THE HEALING POWER OF CAYENNE PEPPER

the complete handbook of cayenne remedies

Patrick Quillin, PhD,RD,CNS

James Direct, Inc.
North Canton, Oh

Published by:

James Direct Inc.
1459 S. Main St.
N. Canton, Ohio 44720
U.S.A.

Printing 12 11 10 9 8 7 6 5 4 3 2 1

First Edition   **Copyright 2008**   **James Direct Inc.**

CONTENTS

Fat reduction
Gas
Headache
Heart disease
Heart arrhythmia
Heat exhaustion
Herbal augmentor
High blood pressure
High cholesterol
Libido
Malnutrition
Mouth sores
Nausea
Obesity
Osteoarthritis
Pain
Pesticide
Pleurisy
Psoriasis
Shingles
Sinusitis
Skin problems
Sore throat
Stress reducer
Stroke
Thyroid problems
Toothache Toxin protection
Ulcers
Urinary tract
Warming effect Worms

Dedication

To the true pioneers in integrative health care: Linus Pauling, PhD; Abram Hoffer, MD, PhD; Adelle Davis; Weston Price, DDS; the Shute brothers, MDs; Max Gerson, MD; Virginia Livingston-Wheeler, MD; and many others. Your courage, independent thinking and brilliance have built a road for the rest of us.

Acknowledgements

A special salute to the many scientists who labor to unravel the mysteries of healing foods, like cayenne, which are found in Nature and have no drug company to champion their cause. Where would we be without your persistence and brilliance?

IMPORTANT NOTICE!!! PLEASE READ!!!
The information and products outlined in this book are designed to be used in conjunction with, not instead of, your doctor's program. If you have an illness, then seek a doctor's care. Do not use this information as sole therapy against any disease. Cayenne is a food supplement and is not intended to diagnose, treat, cure or prevent any disease. This information has not been evaluated by the Food and Drug Administration.

CHAPTER ONE

OVERVIEW AND HIGHLIGHTS
※
IS CAYENNE
A WONDER DRUG?

*Epithets, like pepper, Give zest to what you write; And if
you strew them sparely, They whet the appetite
But if you lay them on too thick, You spoil the matter
quite!*   *Lewis Carroll*

I t is a gift to humanity and a puzzle to scientists.
A "gift" because, next to garlic, it has more
health benefits than any other food/herb on
earth with over 3000
scientific studies to support its
use in preventing and reversing
many common health ailments. A
"puzzle" because it simultaneously
heats and cools, rewards and
torments. "It" is cayenne pepper,
the most widely studied and easily
available of the many hot chili
peppers on earth.

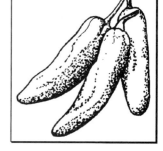

     Some people love it and some people hate it, but
everyone has to respect the impact that this humble little

fruit, cayenne, has had on the history of mankind. It has been used as a weapon, a food, a spice, and an herbal medicine for over 9000 years[1]. Chili peppers, including cayenne, are consumed regularly by over 1.5 billion people each day, or 25% of the world's population, which makes it one of the most popular foods in the world. Chili peppers, also spelled as "chile" or "chilli", may well be the first cultivated food when our "hunter gatherer" ancestors decided to settle down to farming.

The list of ailments that can be improved with the use of cayenne boggles the imagination. From asthma to pain reduction to melting away pounds to preventing heart disease; there are only a handful of "superherbs" on the planet earth that can match cayenne for its versatility, taste, therapeutic value and safety.

The list of enigmas regarding cayenne is impressive:
*   How can it cool you and warm you at the same time?
*   How can it feel like its burning, but actually reduces the pain from burns?
*   How can it hurt so bad when the amateur eats it, yet it helps the body to generate an internal form of morphine-like pleasure?
*   How can it be so selectively good for your body cells while it is viciously lethal to intestinal bacteria and parasite cells?

This book is a complete compilation of valuable facts about cayenne. It just may be the most important book that you ever read.

SOME HISTORY AND DETAILS

NAME CONFUSION

Its not from the country Chile and its not really a pepper, and, much to the dismay of East Indians, hot peppers were first cultivated in the Americas. So who started all of this name confusion? You have to admire the courage, persistence and creative thinking of Christopher Columbus. When he set sail in 1492 in pursuit of peppercorns found along the coast of India, most everyone watching him disappear over the horizon

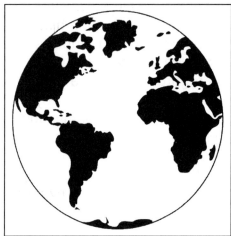

thought that he would fall off the edge of the earth. Instead of sailing over some cataclysmic waterfall or landing in India, Columbus landed in the Caribbean, some 11,000 miles short of his destination. Undaunted, he called the locals "Indians", a name distortion that Native Americans have grappled with ever since; and he called the local "aji" food spices "peppers" to try to please his patrons back home.

Columbus was not looking for gold or real estate, but rather for spices to liven up the otherwise boring menu items consumed by royalty throughout Europe. Remember, in those days, without refrigeration, food began rotting as soon as it was slaughtered or picked, thus spices were more than a hedonistic pleasure, they were necessary to overcome the stench of food that was beginning to decay. Pepper, or Piper nigrum, from the Malabar coast of India was the spice of choice in those days; it was first brought overland to Europe by Chinese and Arab traders. Due to the extraordinary effort of moving pepper, ginger, cinnamon and other spices across 6,000 miles of treacherous land, the cost for these spices in Europe was quite high and only available to royalty.

Columbus found no black peppercorns in his "India", but on his second voyage to the New World, his accompanying physician, Dr. Diego Alvarez Chanca, picked up some of the local spices, then called "aji", which were regularly served by the native Arawak people. In an attempt to please his "venture capitalists" in England, Columbus called the aji "peppers", but the food was initially deemed unfit for consumption by the royal physicians and scientists throughout Europe. Columbus died as an unheralded pauper.

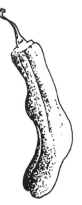

From Europe, the chili plants and seeds were brought around the world by ocean explorers and thrived in many parts of South America, Africa and Asia. It took 50 years before the tomato from America and the potato from the Andes highlands of South America were accepted as a food in Europe. In that same time frame of 50 years, chilis circumnavigated the globe and were grown on every continent but Antarctica. Such was the appeal of this humble little fruit. While we know that the "cradle" of chili cultivation was somewhere in Central or South America, the best guess for its exact location is Bolivia. The hottest pepper in the world is the habanero, grown only in the Yucatan area of Mexico. The Mayan natives there consider the regular consumption of the habanero to be a "rite of passage", which few outsiders can pass.

Later, this aji, or chili pepper was more accurately classified as a fruit belonging to the genus Capsicum annuum, which includes red pepper, anaheim, ancho, cayenne, cherry, chili, green bell pepper, hot pepper, jalapeno, paprika, pimento, piquin and red bell pepper[2]. Tabasco pepper belongs to the Capsicum frutescens genus and the hottest pepper in the world, Habanero, belongs to Capsicum chinense. This Capsicum genus belongs to the family Solanaceae, which includes tomatoes and potatoes. So realize, that as we charge ahead with discussion of "cayenne", that this is only one of many chili peppers, more accurately called Capsicum, that is found throughout the world. What we are really talking about in this book is the incredible healing and pleasurable value of hot chilis from around the world, with the most commonly available and best studied one being cayenne.

It was the Greek spice merchants in the 16th century who decided to end the confusion between black peppers and these "quasi" peppers by calling the red, green and yellow chilis: chili pepper. Hungarians decided to call their prize chilis "paprika". Italians called it "peperone". The English called theirs "red pepper", Germans "Indianifcher pfeffer," the French "poivre de l'Inde", and "mircha" in India. "A rose by any other name is still a rose" and all of these delightful varieties of hot chilis have pleased and healed billions of people for the past 90 centuries.

WHO GROWS IT?

Capsicum plants grow around the world in many climates on many continents. But there are some basic ground rules:

1) the hotter the climate, the hotter the chili

2) the smaller the chili, the hotter the taste.

New Mexico along with parts of Louisiana are the epicenters of chili farming in the United States. Most chilis require an optimal growing temperature of 24 degrees C. (93 F.) with a tolerable temperature range of 32 C. (103 F.) and 15 C. (59 F.). Humidity is a must. Three to five months is the average growing time for most chilis before harvest. There are over 1,700 different

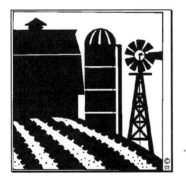 varieties of both wild and culti-vated peppers known[3].

Hungary uses twice as much acreage to grow paprika chilis as tomato plants, pro-ducing over 62,000 tons per year. India produces over 800,000 tons of chilis annually and consumes 95% of it right there at home. The chili growing nations of India, Hungary, China, Pakistan, Mexico, Sri Lanka, Nigeria, Ethiopia, Thailand, and Japan produce over 4 million tons per year[4]. Mexico cultivates the widest assortment of chilis in its 53,000 tons per year, with only a small percentage being the bland bell pepper and nearly all of that going to the United States. The hottest pepper commonly found in American markets is the Jalapeño, grown in Jalapa, Veracruz in Mexico. New Mexico grows around 47,000 tons of chilis annually, leading all American states.

American farmers wishing to diversify their crops may consider the humble chili as a "cash crop", which nets a profit of $1600 per acre, compared to $300 per acre for hay. Meanwhile, the infamous black pepper that Columbus sought, amounts to only 200,000 tons of production per year around the world.

HELPED WIN A NOBEL PRIZE

Dr. Albert Szent-Gyorgyi was a Hungarian scientist doing research in the United States during the 1930s. He was trying to isolate hexuronic acid from the adrenals of cattle. After laboring for years and tediously extracting hexuronic acid from vast quantities of cow adrenal glands, he managed to gather a mere 20 grams (less than an ounce) of pure hexuronic acid from the hundreds of kilograms of adrenals that he had processed.

Then, once back home in Hungary, his wife fed him a paprika chili pepper for dinner. Lacking an appetite, he decided to take the paprika down to his laboratory and see if it had any hexuronic acid. As we now know, chili peppers have more hexuronic acid, or vitamin C, than almost any other food on earth, as much as 500% more vitamin C per gram than an orange. Dr. Szent-Gyorgyi was elated, able to extract enough vitamin C to identify the chemical structure and was awarded the Nobel prize in 1937 for what Time® Magazine then called "the Paprika Prize". Vitamin C has since become one of the more valuable nutrients in human nutrition, since it bolsters the immune system and slows down the aging process.

AS A WEAPON?

When the Spanish Conquistadors were attacking the Mayan and Incan people in Central and South America during the 16th century, one of the few weapons those people had was to burn large mounds of dried chili peppers in the path of the oncoming invaders, which temporarily blinded the advancing soldiers. More recently, 13 shoppers at a mall in San Fernando, California were hospitalized when a fire broke out in a restaurant and then began burning hot chilis. The fumes from these burning chilis acted like spray Mace on the eyes and lungs of the shoppers.

The bite of chili peppers has been used for brutal purposes. The British rubbed hot Bahamian peppers in the eyes of mutinous slaves in the Caribbean region. In 1640, Sir John Parkinson wrote that dogs detested hot peppers, which eventually produced the aerosol pepper sprays carried by postmen and many women today. It is still custom in some regions of Africa to spray water containing hot pepper juice in the eyes of misbehaving children. The U.S. Army considered using chili powder as a non-lethal form of tear gas. The Grebo tribe in Liberia still conduct a sadistic ritual of smearing mashed hot peppers in every orifice of an infant's body as a means of "initiating" the child.

WHAT'S IN IT?

When we arrive at the HEALTH BENEFITS section of this book, you are going to be amazed at the healing properties of cayenne. Therefore, we need to peer inside of this humble little fruit in order to better understand how it may help an alphabet soup of health problems. Bear with me for a minute. There is a purpose to this section.

The "bite" in cayenne is from a compound called "capsaicin", with the family of related compounds called "capsaicinoids" found in hot peppers throughout the world. Chemists call capsaicin "8 methyl N vanillyl 6 none-namide". Capsaicin has a chemical structure very similar to the active ingredient in ginger, both of which have a pungent "bite" and many therapeutic values.

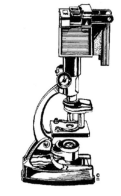

In addition to capsaicin, which we will spend considerable time discussing in the next section, a fresh cayenne chili pepper contains[5]:

```
Water: 9%
Carbohydrate: 54%
Starch: 1%
Protein: 13%
Fiber: 31%
Ash (minerals): 6%
Fat soluble "others": 22%
Vitamin C: 29 mg per 100 grams
Capsaicinoids: 177 micrograms per gram
Beta carotene: 1733 micrograms per gram
Iron: 10 mg per 100 grams
Phosphorus: 356 mg per 100 grams
Calcium: 210 mg per 100 grams
```

The health of Americans is suffering from too much fat and the wrong kind of fat. Chili peppers are both low in fat and contain the right kind of fat: 66% of the fat as linoleic and 5% as linolenic acid, the two essential fats in the diet of humans. Phospholipids are valuable fats that are bound to the mineral phosphorus and make up much of our cell membranes and escort molecules in the blood. In chili peppers, 76% of the phospholipids are lecithin (phosphatidylcholine), which is an extremely valuable nutrient for the heart and brain.

The fabulous rainbow of colors that are found in chili peppers contain thousands of bioflavonoids and carotenoids, which may be partly responsible for the healing properties of cayenne. These natural pigments help chlorophyll in capturing the sun's energy in the process called photosynthesis. Some of these colorful and healthful substances are: beta-carotene, zeaxanthin, cryptoxanthin, violaxanthin, neoxanthin, antheraxanthin, cryptoxanthin, and lutein. Free range chickens eat a wide assortment of these natural pigments and produce eggs with deep reddish orange yolk, which reflects the healthful nutrients in the chicken's diet. Cayenne powder is added to commercial chicken feed to give their egg yolk the healthy color that we look for.

The real "business end" of cayenne is the "bite", which comes from capsaicin. There are varying levels of capsaicin in the multitude of hot peppers found around the world. Capsaicin content ranges from a high of 1.8% in the newly bred Jwala from India to a low of 0.02% found in Hungarian paprika. Topical ointments with capsaicin contain anywhere from 0.025% to 0.075%. Keep this in mind as we later talk about toxicity of cayenne and other chili peppers. Nature never puts much more than 1% of capsaicin in its chili fruits.

MECCA FOR "CHILIHEADS"

Those people who develop a passion for the bite of chili peppers are affectionately called "chiliheads". They will go to any length to get their high from their favorite chili. Zubin Mehta, the famous philharmonic conductor, brings his own hot peppers with him, even to the finest restaurants in the world, where the chef's eagerly greet him and take his peppers into the kitchen to be added gracefully to his meal. The King of Spain plucked a few peppers from Mehta's garden and brought them home for his garden. It was "chiliheads" like these celebrities who spread the hot pepper around the world in only 50 years.

Mrs. Frank Sinatra is an equal fan of hot peppers and carried them with her everywhere as well as grew her own in her California home. Gregory Peck was so enamored at Mrs. Sinatra's flavorful habit, that he too became a chilihead and started his own garden. All U.S. astronauts are provided a "kit" for space travel that includes hot peppers, which wasn't quite good enough for astronaut and chilihead extraordinaire William Lenoir who took a jalapeño with him on a space voyage in 1982.

For chiliheads looking for pilgrimages to the "promised land", there are many regions and countries willing to fight for the title of chili capital. In the U.S., the Rio Grande area of New Mexico and Texas grow the most chilis. Meanwhile, Edmund McIlhenny, developer of the infamous Tabasco® sauce, founded a chili pepper empire on Avery Island, Louisiana in 1862. If you are looking for the world's hottest chili pepper, then buy a ticket to the Yucatan Peninsula of Mexico and dine with the native Mayans. If it is serious hot chilis that you are after, then people in Thailand consume 5 grams daily, twice the amount of Indian chiliheads. If its chili commerce that you are after, then head to Guntur in southeast India, where the planting, harvesting, processing and eating of chilis occupies most of the locals most of the time. Koreans and their kimchi and Chinese Szechwan residents might protest these verdicts, due to their own chili obsessions.

WHAT DOES CAYENNE DO TO THE BODY?

Here's where it starts looking "too good to be true"; but it is true. The whole concept of a simple fruit, like cayenne, generating healing benefits for such a wide assortment of ailments seems a bit preposterous. Until you realize that bread mold was used for centuries in Ayurvedic medicine as an antibiotic before Alexander Fleming isolated the mold extract, penicillin, that specifically kills bacteria. White willow bark was used for centuries by Native American medicine men for treating aches, pains and the flu before a scientist in this century was awarded the Nobel prize for explaining how aspirin (the active ingredient in white willow bark) works.

Curare is an herbal extract that has been used for centuries as a muscle relaxant in the Amazon jungle. The local people apply curare to the tip of a dart, shoot a monkey, and the curare weakens the monkey until it drops out of the tree and becomes dinner. In the past few decades, curare has become a favorite medication for anesthesiologist in the operating room to keep the patient's muscles relaxed.

Ephedra, used as a pure drug to treat asthma, was originally derived from the Chinese herb, Ma Huang. Robitussin® is one of the more common over-the-counter drugs used to loosen mucus, called an expectorant. The active ingredient in Robitussin® is guaifenesin, which is derived from guaiacol, which has the same chemical structure as capsaicin. In fact, one third of all prescription drugs in the United States were derived from a plant compound--just like cayenne.

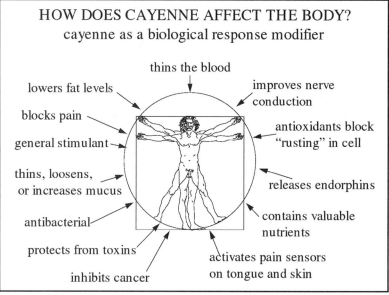

HOW DOES CAYENNE AFFECT THE BODY?
cayenne as a biological response modifier

thins the blood

lowers fat levels

blocks pain

general stimulant

thins, loosens, or increases mucus

antibacterial

protects from toxins

inhibits cancer

improves nerve conduction

antioxidants block "rusting" in cell

releases endorphins

contains valuable nutrients

activates pain sensors on tongue and skin

What is even more amazing is the 3000 plus scientific studies listed in the National Library of Medicine on the health benefits of capsaicin and cayenne. Nearly all research money in America comes from major drug firms, or the National Institutes of Health, which uses 95% of its money to fund drug studies. Drugs are patentable substances, which can be protected against competition, thus improving the chances of making a substantial profit during the 17 year life of the patent. Natural substances, like cayenne, cannot be patented, and hence are of little interest to drug companies, except to create drug analogs (molecules that are similar to the natural molecule but different enough to be patented). The fact that 3000 studies exist on the merits of capsaicin, with no serious drug patron to fund the studies shows how valuable this humble little fruit may be to our future health care system. Imagine how many studies would be done on capsaicin if we invested research dollars based upon a simple formula of risk to benefit to cost of that item.

The lengthy alphabetical listing in the next section regarding the health benefits from cayenne all stem from the basic mechanisms on how it influences the human body:

Thins the blood. My wife and I took a tour of a southern plantation in Louisiana near the Mississippi River. The tour guide told us that the river would sometimes get "too thick to drink and too thin to plow." The same might be said for the blood of the typical American. With too much fat, saturated fat, cholesterol, and sugar in the diet; and not enough fish oil, flax oil, fiber, vitamin E and cayenne--we end up with blood that is sludgy. Imagine how much harder a swimming pool pump would have to work if the pool was filled with yogurt instead of water. That's how much harder your heart has to work to move the sludgy blood that is a product of our lifestyle.

Our bodies are a miraculous network of 60,000 miles of blood vessels with a heart muscle that pumps 55 million gallons of blood over the course of a lifetime to feed all 60 trillion cells in your body. Some blood vessels are so narrow that the blood cells must squeeze down the passageway like a water balloon being forced down a pipe in order to feed the peripheral cells in the outlying regions.

When the blood gets too thick, it cannot fit into tiny capillaries and many cells that rely on this precarious flow of supplies begin to starve for oxygen and nutrients; then start to accumulate waste products and die in their own toxic mess. When the blood gets too thick, the heart must pump harder to get blood to all areas, thus stressing the heart muscle. When the blood gets too thick, the pressure in the vessels goes up, with hypertension being the result. High blood pressure pounds away at delicate capillaries in the brain and kidney and can cause stroke or organ failure. Cayenne can change all of that.

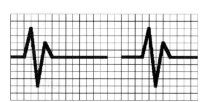 An extremely important research project was conducted by Sukon Visudhiphan, MD, PhD and colleagues in 1981 in which they tested the viscosity of the blood in Americans living in Thailand versus native Thais, who eat copious quantities of hot chilis[6]. Fibrin is the substance in the blood that forms clots when we are cut--something we don't want to happen before we are cut. Fibrinolytic (breaking of fibrin) activity was much higher in the native Thais eating all those spicey chilis. More on this therapeutic activity of cayenne later.

Blocks pain. Certain types of nerves in the human body seem to have receptor sites for capsaicin, kind of like having a keyhole that fits a certain lock. Capsaicin topically applied is able to block the production of substance P (stands for "pain") in nerves without affecting the ability to sense hot, cold or touch[7]. No other substance even comes close to the low 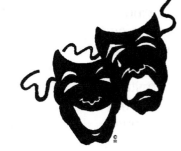 risk analgesic benefits of cayenne in certain conditions.

Enhances nerve conduction. Capsaicin is able to stimulate the conduction of nerve impulses, with the net effect of energizing the nerves, muscles and brain. Given the fact that one of the most common complaints among Americans is fatigue, this should come as welcome news.

Increases mucus flow. Since capsaicin is a mild irritant to mucus membranes, the capsaicin heightens the flow of mucus which flushes out bacteria, virus and debris from the sinuses and lungs. This mildly irritating quality of cayenne seems to put it on the "no-no" list for people with ulcers. Actually researchers find that cayenne, taken in reasonable quantities, may accelerate the healing of ulcers by creating a flow of protective mucus while also directly killing the bacteria Helicobacter pylori that can cause ulcers.

Changes fat metabolism. Capsaicin is able to block the reabsorption of cholesterol in the gut and to slow down the manufacturing of cholesterol in the liver. It also helps to mobilize fats as serum triglycerides to keep them from permanently parking in the liver, which helps to prevent fatty liver. More on this feature of cayenne in later sections.

Antioxidant slows oxidation and aging. After nearly 40 years of research, scientists have generally agreed on the importance of free radicals (a.k.a. reactive oxygen species, pro oxidants) and antioxidants. Free radicals are like little fires that crop up around your body all day every day. Free radicals come from the toxins we inhale, eat and drink (like tobacco and alcohol) and the free radicals that we generate as part of living. These fires can burn up valuable tissue, like the DNA to start cancer, or the cornea of the eye to begin cataracts, or the brain to begin Alzheimers, or the lining of the blood vessels to begin heart disease. Antioxidants are the "fire extinguishers" that put out these free radical fires. In the process of putting out the fire, antioxidants get used up. Hence, there must be a continuous flow of antioxidants into the body to slow down the incessant onslaught of degenerative disease and aging.

Antioxidants include:

⇒ vitamins, like C, E and beta-carotene

⇒ minerals, like selenium

⇒ amino acids, like glutathione

⇒ bioflavonoids, like quercetin from orange peelings

⇒ mixed carotenoids, like lycopenes from tomatoes

⇒ other substances, like chlorophyll from spinach or Coenzyme Q from liver.

There are several known antioxidants in cayenne, including beta-carotene, bioflavonoids and vitamin C; but these do not quite account for the ability of cayenne to slow the aging process and retard the effects of free radicals. Scientists are giving up on trying to find that one "magic bullet" antioxidant, and have realized that a mixture of antioxidants give much better protection against free radical damage[8]. We are only beginning to understand the complexities and importance of antioxidants. Since paprika peppers have already played such an important role in the understanding of antioxidants through the discovery of vitamin C, no doubt there are more antioxidant mystery substances waiting to be uncovered in hot chilis.

Releases endorphins. The reason that a morphine addict can get "high" off of his drug is that the human brain has receptor sites for heroine and morphine, more accurately known as endorphins ("endo" for inside us and "orphin" for morphine). The body uses these "rivers of pleasure" to reduce pain during childbirth and major cuts and burns, while also letting endorphins flow when we are doing something that we enjoy. When we eat cayenne, we feel an initial burning sensation, though it doesn't really burn anything. The body thinks that a burn has occurred and lets a little endorphin flow to soothe the wound. People who eat hot chilis on a regular basis actually become addicted to the endorphin flow, not unlike long distance runners who get high from their endorphin flow.

Valuable nutrients. High in protein, fiber, vitamin C, bioflavonoids, mixed carotenoids and some essential fatty acids; cayenne is a "nutrient dense" food, not unlike Uranium is an energy-dense radioactive element. No doubt, there are as-yet undetermined nutrients lurking within the shadows of cayenne that add to its healing value.

Inhibits cancer. Eating too much hot peppers was once considered a mild risk for getting cancer. We now find that capsaicin can inhibit the transformation of cells that gear up toward full blown cancer. Capsaicin was able to block the generation of cancer from one of the more cancer-causing substances on earth, aflatoxins.

Protects stomach from alcohol and aspirin. While many people labor under the misconception that cayenne irritates the stomach, and it can in higher doses, actually aspirin is one of the more lethal compounds on the stomach. Aspirin causes microscopic bleeding in the lining of the stomach, which kills 3,300 older Americans each year from hemorrhaging. Alcohol is a milder irritant on the stomach lining. Cayenne has been shown in scientific studies to protect the lining of the stomach from potential damage caused by aspirin and alcohol.

Kills microorganisms. Cayenne has been shown to be one of the more potent and selectively toxic substance known in killing bacteria, viruses, worms, and parasites.

Based upon the above list of actions on the human body, in the next section you will read a very impressive list of health benefits from cayenne.

SUPERFOODS & SUPERHERBS

There are many nourishing foods among the 20,000 edible plants and thousands of edible animals and insects on earth. Yet, there are only a handful of "superfoods" which are so nutrient-dense that they merit inclusion in your diet on a regular basis. "Nutrient density" refers to the amount of vitamins, minerals, protein, fiber and conditionally essential nutrients (like lipoic acid, carnitine and EPA) found per 100 calories of that food. So, for instance, the nutrient density of broccoli is much better than for chocolate cake; liver is better than prime rib, 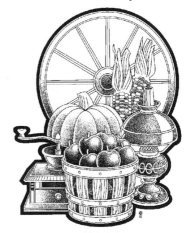 spinach is better than iceberg lettuce, and so on. Based upon these guidelines there are several foods that should be eaten often by nearly everyone (unless you have an allergy to that food) to achieve optimum health:

SUPERFOODS

-hot chili peppers, including cayenne
-garlic
-dark green leafy vegetables, including spinach, collards, beet greens
-tomatoes
-whole grains, like oats, wheat and rice
-legumes, like soy and garbanzo beans
-fruits rich in enzymes, including kiwi, papaya, and pineapple

-cold water ocean fish, including salmon, tuna, halibut, anchovies

-cruciferous vegetables, including cauliflower, brussel sprouts, broccoli

There is another set of "superherbs" that are so potent and so non-toxic that they need to be included on a regular basis to ensure optimal health. These herbs stimulate "host defense mechanisms" for a stronger immune system, more balanced blood glucose levels, healthier prostaglandins and more.

SUPERHERBS

-hot chili peppers, including cayenne

-garlic

-echinacea

-ginger

-turmeric

-ginseng

-goldenseal

-astragalus

-green tea (Camellia sinensis)

-licorice

Note that only two items on the planet earth qualify in both "superfood" and "superherb" category: hot chilis and garlic. For more on garlic, see my book *HONEY, GARLIC AND VINEGAR.*

HOW MUCH IS ENOUGH?
CAN YOU EAT TOO MUCH?

Nothing in life is perfectly safe. Over the years many Americans have died from electrocution while using a hair dryer and standing in a bathtub full of water. That doesn't mean that we should ban hair dryers, which are now quite safe. Thousands of Americans die every year from the hemorrhaging effects caused by aspirin, one of the most widely used and most valuable over-the-counter medications. No one has died from the use of cayenne, although some novices accidentally biting into the infamous habanero firecracker might briefly wish for a peaceful

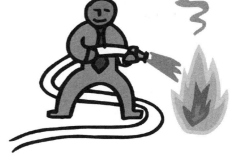

death. On a risk to benefit to cost ratio, cayenne is extremely safe and useful at improving the health for most people.

As with anything in life, you want the right amount. Too much cayenne will not only send your mouth into a 4 alarm fire drill and burn you at the other end, but may end up doing more harm than good. Cayenne is a mildly irritating substance on the gastro-intestinal tract. Cayenne should be avoided by people with hemorrhoids, since the "burn at both end" slogan at many chili festivals will antagonize hemorrhoids[9]. Small amounts of cayenne increase the flow of gastric secretions, which improves digestion, appetite and elimination. Too much cayenne and you have stomach irritation, nausea, maldigestion of nutrients and possibly diarrhea. The novice is going to find that cayenne requires an adaptation period. Build up to eating a reasonable level. See the section at the end of this chapter on "getting started". Do not eat cayennes to demonstrate your macho ability to withstand pain. Too much or too little exercise, sunshine and cayenne are all bad for you. Good judgment needs to be used in finding the right amount of cayenne for you.

Cayenne should never be rubbed on an open wound. Do not inhale cayenne powder or serious spasms of coughing and sneezing will follow. Do not get any hot peppers in your eyes. If applied to the skin in high concentrations (greater than 1% solution) it can create serious irritation spots. Originally, there was some concern that hot chilis taken in excess could increase the risk of stomach cancer; however more research points to moderate use of cayenne as a potent protector against cancer. See the section following on "cancer prevention". All of the above precautions regarding the use of cayenne should be heeded, yet realize that you don't need to go to the emergency room if you get some cayenne in your eyes. Just flush it out and wait for the "burn" to subside. Cayenne may be occasionally painful, but it is not poisonous. Cayenne is found on the Generally Recognized As Safe (GRAS) list by the Food and Drug Administration[10].

AMERICA'S HEALTH CARE MELTDOWN WHY WE NEED CAYENNE

America spends over $1 trillion each year on what we euphemistically call "health care", which is more "disease maintenance" than anything else. We spend twice the money per capita as any other nation on earth for health care. And our "health state of the union" is less than spectacular:

-50 million Americans have high blood pressure
-More than 1/3 of us die from cardiovascular disease and one fourth from cancer, both diseases were relatively unknown prior to the 20th century
-70 million have sleep problems
-50 million have regular headaches
-55 billion aspirin are consumed yearly
-9 million Americans are alcoholics
-64% are overweight
-44 million have mental illness
-9.6 million older adults each year suffer drug-induced side effects, including 659,000 hospitalizations and 163,000 with memory loss

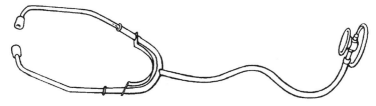

When the doctor sets a broken bone, he or she does not heal the patient, but rather sets in place the tissue so that Nature can heal us from within. Same thing happens in stitching up a cut, or when you recovered from your last bought with the flu. The only way you stay well or heal from a health challenge is by nourishing that "God-given life force" within us. When we stop trying to change natural biochemical laws, then we will find a quantum leap in our health and improved results at the doctor's office.

America has among the highest incidences in the world for heart disease, cancer, diabetes, mental illness, osteoporosis, and other diseases. We have a worse infant survival record than many European countries and Canada.

MALNUTRITION IN AMERICA
THE GREAT NUTRITION ROBBERY

America is the most agriculturally productive nation in the history of the world. We grow enough food in this country to feed ourselves, to make half of us overweight, to throw away enough food to feed 50 million people daily, to ship food overseas as a major export, and to store enough food in government surplus bins to feed Americans for a year if all farmers quit today. With so much food available, how can Americans be mal-nourished? The simple answer is: poor food choices.

People in Western Society chose their food based upon taste, cost, convenience and psychological gratification--thus ignoring the main reason that we eat, which is to provide our body with the raw materials to grow, repair and fuel our cells. We take Nature's elegantly designed nutritious foods and:

⇒ use drugs, hormones, and antibiotics to raise animals faster, while spraying 1.2 billion pounds of pesticides over our food crops

⇒ fail to properly fertilize the soil with organic matter

and trace minerals, which creates mineral-poor crops
⇨ remove vitamins, minerals, and fiber during extensive food processing
⇨ add over 2800 Food and Drug Administration approved additives, including salt, fat, sugar, and unsafe food additives, like saccharin and MSG
⇨ dramatically increase the cost of the food, which compounds the problems for the poor.

The fact is: the nutrients were in that food for a very good reason. When we tamper with the food supply, we usually wreak havoc on the food's nutritional content. The most commonly eaten foods in America are white bread, coffee and hot dogs, which have little to offer the body. Based upon our food abundance and affluence, Americans could be the best nourished nation on record. But we are far from it.

In the late 1930s, Dr. Weston Price, a dentist, and his wife, Monica, who was a nurse, were intrigued by the possible link between diet and health. In true "Indiana Jones" adventuresome fashion, they travelled the world logging over 100,000 miles on primitive aircraft to investigate 17 different cultures[11]. What they found was startling to scientists then. The more refined (read: adulterated) the food supply, the worse the health of the people. Those people who ate their ancestral diet had excellent health, teeth structure, energy, and appearance. Those who deviated from their ancestral diet suffered everything from mild symptoms, such as acne, skin and hair problems, and poor dental formation to the severest forms of mental retardation and even paralysis.

Another group of researchers from Emory University in Atlanta followed up on Dr. Price's work in 1988 and found similar results. They stated that the "paleolithic" diet was very different from our current refined diet, and that difference may contribute to many of our ailments[12]. Our ancestors, the hunter and gatherers, ate a superior diet and enjoyed superior health. See the chart below which compares our modern diet to that of our hunter gatherer ancestral era.

MOST POPULAR GROCERY ITEMS IN AMERICA

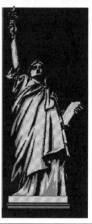

1. Marlboro cigarettes
2. Coke Classic
3. Pepsi Cola
4. Kraft processed cheese
5. Diet Coke
6. Campbell's soup
7. Budweiser beer
8. Tide detergent
9. Folger's coffee
10. Winston cigarettes

from "1992 Top Ten Almanac"
by Michael Robbins

Overwhelming evidence from government surveys of 200,000 Americans and numerous respected universities shows that many Americans are low in their intake of:

-VITAMINS: A, D, E, C, B-6, riboflavin, folacin, pantothenic acid

-MINERALS: calcium, potassium, magnesium, zinc, iron, chromium, selenium; and possibly molybdenum and vanadium.

-MACRONUTRIENTS: fiber, complex carbohydrates,

plant protein, special fatty acids (EPA, GLA, ALA), clean water

Meanwhile, we also eat alarmingly high amounts of: fat, salt, sugar, cholesterol, alcohol, caffeine, food additives and toxins.

This combination of too much of the wrong things along with not enough of the right things has created epidemic proportions of degenerative diseases in this country. The Surgeon General, Department of Health and Human Services, Centers for Disease Control and Prevention, National Academy of Sciences, American Medical Association, American Dietetic Association, and most other major public health agencies agree that diet is a major contributor to our most common health problems, including cancer and heart disease.

The typical American diet is high in fat while being low in fiber and vegetables. "Meat, potatoes, and gravy" is what many of my cancer patients lived on for decades. Data collected by the United States Department of Agriculture from over 11,000 Americans showed that on any given day:

-41 percent did not eat any fruit

-82 percent did not eat cruciferous vegetables

-72 percent did not eat vitamin C-rich fruits or vegetables

-80 percent did not eat vitamin A-rich fruits or vegetables

-84 percent did not eat high fiber grain food, like bread or cereal

The human body is incredibly resilient, which sometimes works to our disadvantage. No one dies on the first cigarette inhaled, or the first drunken evening, or the first decade of unhealthy eating. We misconstrue the fact that we survived this ordeal to mean we can do it forever. Not so. Malnutrition can be blatant, as the starving babies in third world countries. Malnutrition can also be much more slow and subtle; first bringing the vague symptoms of chronic fatigue, constipation, mood swings, poor wound recovery, and frequent colds; followed by a decade of struggling with incontinence, poor memory, pain in the chest, poor digestion, and visual problems. Malnutrition in America is a progressive and silent saboteur from within the body, not an instant knockout punch.

It was the Framingham study done by Harvard University that proclaimed: "Our way of life is related to our way of death." While many Americans are overfed, the majority are also poorly nourished. The typical American, statistically speaking, is overweight, has six colds per year, is regularly plagued with lethargy, mild depression, and constipation, gets dentures by age 45, begins a marked decline in function and vitality by age 50, and dies in their 60s or 70s from heart disease or cancer. Another scientist has stated the problem more bluntly: "We are digging our graves with our teeth." A return to healthier foods, including cayenne, would make a marked difference in the health of Americans. But remember, it is always best to adopt a healthier lifestyle rather than relying on one "magic bullet" drug or food (even cayenne) to rescue you from a health challenge. A healthier lifestyle includes moderate exercise, a good diet, rest and meditation and avoidance of toxins.

USE AND ABUSE OF MODERN MEDICINE

"Let food be your medicine and let medicine be your food." Hippocrates, father of modern medicine 400 BC

America has the most expensive and technologically advanced health care system in the world. For acute critical care, no medical system in the world can match ours. Yet, oftentimes we fight the symptoms of degenerative diseases with drugs and surgery in a futile losing battle, when the real answer to the patient's health problems might have been something as simple as diet improvement, or gentle herbal healers like cayenne, or a sympathetic ear. Think of a sink overflowing with a mess of water all over the floor. Our medical system spends an incredible amount of time and money trying to wipe up the mess on the floor when the easiest solution is to turn off the faucet that produces the diseases.

Dr. Christiaan Barnard, the pioneering heart transplant surgeon, claimed that the greatest advancement in health care in the last 500 years came from, not a drug or surgical procedure, but the invention of the indoor flushing toilet, thus eliminating the many plagues caused by contaminated water supplies. The World Health Organization has reported that 70-80% of the world's population uses herbs and foods as their primary healing instruments, many of which are in jeopardy of being lost as the tropical rain forests disappear. Hippocrates, the Greek father of modern medicine told us 2400 years ago "Let food be your medicine and medicine be your food" and "...in nature there is strength."

Throughout the world and recorded history, natural

healing agents were the main tools of the physician, with herbs serving as the favored medicines. Avicenna was an Arab herbalist who lived in the 11th century and travelled extensively throughout the known world to catalog the medical uses of herbs. He eventually wrote 100 books on this subject, culminating in his 1 million word tome: CANON OF MEDICINE. This book was considered a standard for medical education throughout Europe and Asia until the 17th century. Hippocrates, the father of modern medicine, used cayenne in several of his healing herbal remedies.

The big shift in medical outlook began with a Swiss physician, Theophrastus von Hohenheim, who became discontent in the early 16th century with his training and began wandering Europe. While in the mines in Italy, Hohenheim was intrigued by the refining of minerals. He took this knowledge and began using mercury, a known poisonous metal, to treat his patients. He further dabbled in the use of strong minerals for medicines. His methods were widely criticized and he died after being tossed from a window by his adversaries while only 50 years old.

By 1928, Alexander Fleming had taken penicillin from bread mold and injected it into a patient with an infection. The recovery process was astoundingly quick and the era of antibiotics was born. By the end of World War II, the development of chemicals was coming faster than they could be cataloged or tested for safety. The chemical age was born, and with it came the mixed blessings of miracle chemicals and the immoral contamination of our planet. In the 1950s, Jonas Salk brought us the polio vaccine, and helped to end one of the worst scourges of mankind.

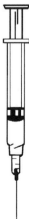

There is a difference between using our knowledge to improve our lot and abusing our knowledge through ego to worsen our lot. Drugs and surgery have their places in the healing arts, especially as short term fixes to get an acutely ill patient through a crisis phase. There are times when no other form of healing will work. But when we rely on these invasive therapies to heal a problem which can only be healed by following natural biochemical laws, we end up worse off. We need to be more restrained with medical therapies and more liberal with natural healing therapies, like cayenne. The intelligent combination would leave us with astoundingly good health. First, try the "cell restoration" therapies which include cayenne, and only as a last resort should we use the symptom-treating therapies of drugs and surgery.

I have worked with many patients who were defying all of Nature's laws: poor food, smoking, no exercise, stress, and a body loaded with toxins. Without a thought for changing this semi-suicidal lifestyle, the doctor will put the patient on an endless array of prescription drugs, which all have dastardly side effects, until the patient eventually develops a really serious disease, like cancer. We arrogantly assume that drugs can reverse the abuse caused by decades of poor nutrition and toxic burden. We are not respecting the laws of nature.

Cayenne is one of Nature's truly remarkable healing forces. But cayenne alone cannot negate the influence of living off of Pop Tarts®, Oreos®, cigarettes, TV and stress. Start incorporating an overall healthy lifestyle if you want to derive maximum benefits from the use of cayenne.

ANTIDOTES FOR THE "SINS" OF AMERICAN EATING

There was a report published in the *Journal of the National Cancer Institute* which found that the more pizza men ate, the lower was their risk for prostate cancer[13]. Not that pizza is good for you, with high fat cheese, white flour crust and lots of fat added. But, the tomato sauce is one of the richest sources of lycopenes, which are such a powerful healing factor that lycopenes, even with the rest of the unhealthy baggage from pizza, can reduce the risk for one of the more common killers among American men.

Scientists have found a similar "antidote" effect with red wine. Although the French eat as much fat as Americans, and have equally disastrous lifestyles, their regular use of red wine with its healing bioflavonoids has been shown in numerous studies to neutralize the otherwise damaging effects of a not-so-healthy lifestyle.

Garlic can do similar magic. You can commit many errors in your diet, yet include garlic and still have a lower risk for many disease. Cayenne is in this magical "antidote" category. Studies have shown that cayenne can reduce circulating levels of fat and cholesterol in the blood after a high fat meal. You can do many things wrong in your diet, but do a few very important things right and still come out ahead. I believe that Americans are dying more from what we are NOT eating rather than what we are eating. Add garlic, cayenne and tomatoes to an otherwise marginal nutrient intake, and you can neutralize many of the "sins" of the typical American diet.

HOW "HOT" IS HOT?

Based upon the modern 0-10 "heat intensity" rating system, here's how some chilis from around the world rate for "fire power"[14]:

HEAT-CHILIS	COUNTRY GROWN
1-Hungarian sweet chili	east Europe, California
1-Pimento	Hungary, Spain, Calif
3-Anaheim (green, red)	southwestern USA
3-Poblana (green & red)	central Mexico
4-Chawa	Yucatan, Mexico
4-Chilaca	Central Mexico
4-New Mexico	southwest US
5-Guero	southwest US, n. Mexico
5-Jalapeño	Mexico, southwest US
5-De Agua	central Mexico
6-Huachinango	central Mexico
6-Santa Fe Grande	southwest US, n. Mexico
6-Dutch	Holland
6-Fresno	southwest US
7-Korean	Japan, Korea, California
7-Manzana	Central America
7-Peter Pepper	Texas, Louisiana
7-Rocotillo	South America
7-Serrano	southwest US, Mexico
7-Thai	southeast Asia
7-Aji	Peru
7-Amatista	South America
7-Fiesta	north Mexico, Louisiana
8-Peruvian	South America
8-Tepin	Central & South America
9-Jamaican Hot	Caribbean
9-Macho (green & red)	Mexico
9-Scotch Bonnet	Cent.America, Caribbean
9-Tabasco	Louisiana, Cent. America
10-Habanero	Yucatan

Methods of measuring the heat index of chilis has become a complicated process. The Aztecs had 6 categories of heat value for their chili peppers: hot, very hot, very very hot, brilliant hot, extremely hot, and run-away hot. This method worked for the Aztecs, yet for centuries, spice merchants around the world grappled with some way of describing the heat value of the chili peppers being sold to their customers. Finally, in 1912, Wilbur L. Scoville, a pharmacist at the Detroit pharmaceutical firm of Parke-Davis™ (now part of Warner-Lambert™) devised a system using the human tongue to detect dilutions of chili extracts. His rating scale went from zero for bell peppers to 300,000 Scoville units for the revered habanero. A more current method uses a zero (bell pepper) to ten (habanero) system.

In your basic well-stocked American grocery store, you should be able to find the following hot chilis: Poblano, green and red Jalapeño, Habanero, Serrano, Tomatillos, Anaheim, Yellow peppers, and dry peppers.

HOW TO GET STARTED WITH CAYENNE

For the uninitiated, hot chilis may seem like a daunting prospect, having tried a chili at a family picnic, then chugging a glass of cold beverage to try to put out the fire. There are many chilis that are grown around the world. If you want to become a connoisseur on chilis, then consult the appendix for mail order companies who will sell you the most exotic chili, either dried or as a seed to plant in your garden.

For the rest of us who want a little of the cayenne "bite" and all of the cayenne health benefits, start slow. The easiest "entry level" cayenne product is:

1) Tablet form of cayenne. Heat units (HU, or Scoville units) of 40,000 is adequate to get some health benefits. Take 1 to 2 capsules with lunch and dinner. Unless you have an uncommonly strong stomach, do not take capsules of cayenne at breakfast. Mixing cayenne with ginger and guar gum (seaweed) seems to tame some of the fire in cayenne without neutralizing the health benefits. There are "cool" forms of cayenne capsules sold in your health food store. You may eventually venture your way up to the major leagues with the 100,000 heat unit cayenne capsules. Dollar for dollar, you cannot beat the health benefits of taking a few capsules of cayenne daily.

2) Powdered cayenne sprinkled on your food. Use it with or instead of salt for seasoning. Buy chili powder at your grocery store or Spike® brand cayenne pepper (from Gayelord Hauser, Box 9398, Milwaukee, WI 53209) at your health food store. The Spike® brand is not irradiated, which is an advantage. Since chilis grow best in hot humid Third World countries where regulations on pesticides and irradiation are virtually non-existent, I find comfort in buying cayenne and other herbs that are, hopefully, organically grown, or at the least have not been irradiated.

3) Salsa. There are many delicious salsas sold at your local grocery store. Try a few different brands. Most of them will rate the heat value with a thermometer on the side of the label, to give you some forewarning about the "bite" of their product. Mexicans, Indians, Thais, Koreans and other nationalities use their own form of hot sauce on nearly every food eaten.

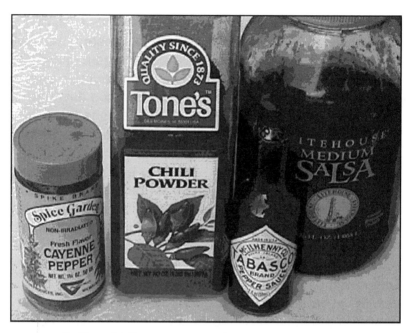

4) Food. There are a few recipes later in this book that give you some ideas on how to incorporate cayenne and other hot peppers into your regular eating pattern. Start slow. Experts tell us that the best way to "put out the fire" from too much hot chilis is to eat dairy products, like yogurt, or bread, or some sugar or ginger, and of course, lots of cool water. You may wish to subscribe to *Chile Pepper* magazine (1-800-ZESTY-ME) for many more ideas on how to enjoy the flavor and health benefits of cayenne.

MY OWN "DANCE" WITH CAYENNE

The ancestral Irish diet does not use much spices. In college I was introduced to the tempestuous and tantalizing treats of hot Mexican food. I was hooked. Though my palate and stomach do not tolerate as much cayenne as many chiliheads, I enjoy the stuff.

If you find no pleasure in a good hot salsa, but still wish to enjoy the health benefits from cayenne, then I suggest taking one or two 40,000 heat unit cayenne capsules with each meal.

Cayenne has helped to clear up my sinuses, giving me more fresh air. Cayenne has improved my physical and mental energy levels and even helped to speed the healing of an occasionally sensitive stomach. From a personal and scientific standpoint, I heartily endorse the frequent use of cayenne for almost anyone.

ENDNOTES

[1]. Cordell, GA, et al., Annals of Pharmacotherapy, vol.27, p.330, Mar.1993

[2]. Palevitch, D., et al., Journal of Herbs & Spices, vol.3, no.2, p.55, 1995

[3]. Foster, S., HERBAL RENAISSANCE, p.63, Gibbs Smith, Salt Lake City, 1984

[4]. Naj, A., PEPPERS, p.17, Vintage Books, NY, 1993

[5]. Govindarajan, VS, et al., CRC Critical Reviews in Food Science and Nutrition, vol.22, no.2, p.108, 1991

[6]. Visudhiphan, S., et al., American Journal Clinical Nutrition, vol.35, p.1452, June 1982

[7]. Colpaert, FC, et al., Life Sciences, vol.32, p.1827, 1983

[8]. Chen, H, et al., Free Radical Biology Medicine, vol.16, p.437, 1994

[9]. Mindell, E., EARL MINDELLS HERB BIBLE, p.63, Simon & Schuster, NY, 1992

[10]. Murray, MT, HEALING POWER OF HERBS, p.76, Prima, Rocklin, CA 1995

[11]. Price, WA, NUTRITION AND PHYSICAL DEGENERATION, Keats, New Canaan, 1945

[12]. Eaton, SB, et al., PALEOLITHIC PRESCRIPTION, Harper, NY, 1988

[13]. Giovannucci, E., et al., Journal National Cancer Institute, vol.87, p.1767, 1995

[14]. Heinerman, J., HEALTH BENEFITS OF CAYENNE, p.43, Keats, New Canaan, CT 1997

CHAPTER TWO

HEALTH BENEFITS OF CAYENNE

Acne. See "skin problems" below.

Allergies. One of the most common symptoms in the world is upper respiratory allergic responses – sneezing, itchy eyes, runny or plugged up nose, wheezing and coughing. Cayenne may help. Capsaicin acts as an antagonist to the kinins and tachykinins that trigger allergic and asthmatic responses. Take 2 capsules of 40,000 heat unit cayenne powder with lunch and dinner. Results should begin within a week.

Angina. Angina is a severe pain in the chest region that basically is caused by the heart muscles being starved for oxygen and nutrients. In 2001, 931,000 Americans died of cardiovascular disease, including 502,000 from heart attack or the later stages of angina (called ischemic heart disease[1]) People who have been through serious angina describe it as a "knife stabbing me right in the heart" followed by the "weight of an elephant sitting on my chest". These are serious signs of heart problems and must be treated with immediate medical attention. Patients who suffer from chronic angina get to experience the pinnacle of miracle drugs in nitroglycerin. Within seconds after placing the nitroglycerin under the tongue, the blood vessels in the heart region begin to dilate and allow some oxygen to reach the starved muscles on the other side of the blockage.

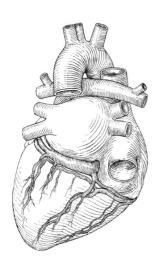

Cayenne can help. Capsaicin triggers the release of a substance called CGRP (calcitonin gene related peptide) which is a potent dilator of the blood vessels that surround the heart[2]. As you work with your doctor, add cayenne to your health regimen, preferably 1-2 capsules of cayenne powder with lunch and dinner. Cayenne will not reduce the effectiveness of any heart medications and may begin to change the under-lying causes of the angina, which drugs never do.

Since the active ingredient in cayenne, capsaicin, is easily dissolved in an alcohol solution, you can prepare a special remedy for angina that has been used by many famous herbalists. In a glass jar with a tight fitting lid, mix one ounce of dried cayenne peppers in with a pint of vodka or gin. Shake several times daily for 2 weeks, then strain this mixture through cheesecloth. Twice daily in between meals, take 6 drops of this tincture either under the tongue or diluted in a glass of water.

Appetite/anorexia. For people with a poor appetite, cayenne may be able to help. Cayenne stimu-lates the gastro-intestinal tract, to help increase the flow of gastric juices (hydrochloric acid and digestive enzymes) along with stimulating the muscles in the GI region to move the food more speedily along--thus making the stomach empty sooner. For speed-eating Americans, you may find that this normally positive effect of cayenne can work against you. Many people report that if they eat too fast and include cayenne in the meal, then they overeat. Slow down your eating so that a meal lasts at least 25 minutes, otherwise the stomach does not have time to send signals to the brain that the stomach is full and the food intake should cease.

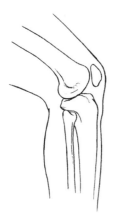

Arthritis. Over 2.1 million Americans suffer from rheumatoid arthritis so severe that it requires medical attention. More than 70 million Americans have some degree of some form of arthritis. Rheumatoid arthritis usually involves an inflammation, thickening and eventually an erosion of the bone ending connective tissue. Osteoarthritis involves the dissolving of the spongy cartilage that cushions the pounding between bone endings. Cayenne to the rescue. Topical application of the more dilute 0.025% capsaicin ointment was able to provide substantial pain relief in patients with both osteo and rheumatoid arthritis within 4 weeks[3]. Another study found good results with capsaicin ointment in osteoarthritis, but no improvement in grip strength, swelling and morning stiffness[4]. In that same study, Drs. McCarthy and McCarty did not find improvements in rheumatoid arthritis from capsaicin. In another study, more than 80% of the patients using the capsaicin ointment felt improvement in morning stiffness and other arthritis-related symptoms, with only 55% of the placebo group feeling relief. There are numerous studies now showing the benefits in reducing pain for arthritis patients. One animal study even showed that capsaicin reduced the swelling from rheumatoid arthritis[5]. During pain response, Substance P is produced in the nerve endings near the joints. Substance P can cause a deterioration in the cartilage surrounding a joint, which means that people should not ignore the pain associated with arthritis, because of this self-perpetuating downward cycle instigated by Substance P. All of this can be helped by capsaicin ointment. See the section "pain" for more information.

Asthma. Asthma can be caused by poor diet (especially low intake of vitamin C and magnesium), stress, air pollution, overexertion in exercise, pollen, ragweed and food allergies. In some of these causes, cayenne can help. Capsaicin seems to be a potent antagonist to several compounds (kinins and tachykinins) which trigger bronchial constriction. The net effect is that regular consumption of cayenne or taking cayenne supplements may help to open the bronchial passageways for asthma sufferers. Take 1-2 capsules of cayenne powder with lunch and dinner. Dr. Jim Duke, a world-famous herbal specialist formerly with the United States Department of Agriculture, told a *USA Today*™ reporter that he cured an asthma attack while in the Costa Rican jungle by sipping a mixture of a pinch of dried cayenne pepper in a glass of hot chocolate.

Baldness. Remember, baldness is mostly a genetic condition. However, for those people who are going bald due to poor circulation in the scalp region, cayenne working as a potent vasodilator may help. Take 2 capsules of 40,000 heat unit cayenne powder with lunch and dinner. If you really want to accelerate the blood supply to the scalp, then mix the powdered contents from 2 cayenne capsules into a small container of pure aloe vera gel. Stir thoroughly. Apply this cayenne mixture to the scalp at bedtime, then wash off in the morning shower.

Bruises & sprains. Cayenne, when applied topically, is able to exhaust the nerve endings of their Substance P (for pain). Cayenne ointment will eventually reduce pain without the use of dangerous drugs, like Tylenol®, or addictive drugs, like codeine. See the sections for "pain" and "osteoarthritis" for more information.

Cancer prevention. While there have been some conflicting reports in this area, it is clear that moderate use of cayenne is cancer protective, while excessive use of chilis may be counterproductive. In one study of Mexicans who ate lots of hot chilis, there was a noticeable increase in the incidence of stomach cancer[6]. To test the theory that capsaicin causes cancer, scientists painted capsaicin on the backs of shaved animals, then applied one of the most potent cancer-causing agents known (DMBA from tobacco smoke) to the skin, with a result of no tumors formed[7]. Other researchers found that cayenne used regularly lowers the incidence of cancer and seems to block the downhill spiral of initiation and promotion that begins cancer[8]. Now, there is an entire series of scientific articles showing that capsaicin prevents the cancer that would have formed from exposure to benzopyrenes (found in overcooked foods), aflatoxin (found in moldy grains and legumes), and tobacco nitrosamines. The conclusions from researchers who are very savvy on foods and cancer: "Although a minute amount of capsaicin displays few or no deleterious effects, heavy ingestion of the compound has been associated with necrosis (death of tissue), ulceration and even carcinogenesis." In other words, if a little hot chilis is good, then more is not better.

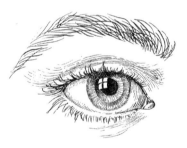

Cataracts. Cataracts involve the loss of transparency in the lens of the eye. Cataract surgery is one of the most common procedures done in American clinics and hospitals, costing Medicare billions of dollars annually. Cataract sufferers liken their problem to "trying to read after smearing Vaseline jelly on your glasses." Cayenne is rich in a collection of bioflavonoids that have been implicated in maintaining healthy vision. Fresh hot chilis (not the dried powder or capsules) are a rich source of vitamin C, which is a potent antioxidant that can slow down the free radical destruction that creates cataracts. Cayenne is also a potent vasodilator, which the lens of the eye can use, given the limited circulation available to that very unusual tissue. All in all, regular use of cayenne may reduce the risk of developing cataracts.

Clogged arteries. See "high cholesterol" and "heart disease" sections.

Colds and flu. If you add up all the amazing effects that cayenne has on the body, it becomes obvious why cayenne has been used for centuries to shorten the severity and duration of colds. Cayenne increases the flow of mucus, which washes away the invading viruses. Cayenne dilates blood vessels to speed the delivery of healing immune factors to the site of infection. As a "beginners" approach to using cayenne for your cold, take 2 capsules of at least 40,000 heat unit cayenne powder with lunch and dinner. For the more advanced followers of cayenne, make a hot tea to gargle with: into 1 cup of warm water mix 2 capsules of 40,000+ heat unit cayenne powder. Swish this fluid around your mouth and gargle. If its too painful, then try half the cayenne powder. Do this 1-3 times daily to help shorten the severity and duration of your colds. Take cayenne supplements and eat cayenne daily to help prevent colds.

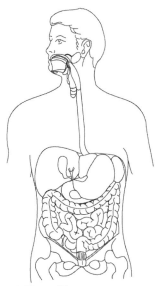

Constipation.

Constipation is one of the more common complaints among Americans. Given our low fiber, low fluid intake along with too much sugar, meat, cheese, and fat; it should not be surprising that the most commonly shoplifted item from American pharmacies is Preparation H, for hemorrhoids. Cayenne increases the flow of juices in the intestinal tract, which helps to speed the food through the GI tract. At moderate intake, hot chilis will encourage regularity. At a higher intake, chilis can cause diarrhea and irritation of the colo-rectal region, hence the slogan at many a chili fest: "Burns at both ends." Obviously, we are looking for healthy and daily bowel elimination, not diarrhea or irritation of hemorrhoids.

Cooling effects. Cayenne is a potent vasodilator. As it opens up the blood vessels near the surface and causes sweating, it creates an initial warming sensation, but is actually bringing the body's internal heat to the surface to be dissipated. Cayenne is regularly consumed by natives of hot humid climates to help them better tolerate the oppressive heat of the tropics. Animal research indicates that cayenne actually triggers the hypothalamus of the brain to cool the body[9]. Just when you think you are fully understanding the breadth of cayenne's healing abilities, then you notice it will also do the opposite. See the "warming effect" section below.

Cough. With its stimulating effect and mild irritation on the mucus membranes, cayenne helps the body to expel whatever is creating the cough. DO NOT breath cayenne powder. Using hot chilis or cayenne capsules will provide support (called an expectorant) in helping the lungs to expel dust, viruses and debris. Dr. Jane Guiltinan of Bastyr University in Seattle has found good success for relieving coughs by mixing: 1 teaspoon of salt, 1/4 teaspoon of cayenne powder and the juice of a half lemon in 4 ounces of warm water. Gargle with this solution as long as you can tolerate it, then spit it out. Do not swallow.

Diabetes. Diabetes mellitus is a common condition of abnormal blood glucose regulation. The name literally means "sweetness running through" since diabetics end up dumping substantial amounts of sugar in their urine, even though the cells of the body are being starved for sugar. Inadequate insulin production, or insulin resistance are common problems. Obesity often compounds diabetes. In 2000, diabetes contributed to 213,000 deaths due to complications such as heart disease, infection, gangrene and kidney failure.
There are several ways that cayenne can help diabetics:
1) as a vasodilator to increase circulation to the peripheral tissue which often gets starved in diabetics and results in poor circulation and gangrene
2) lowering blood glucose levels[10]
3) applied topically to reduce the common pain

from diabetic neuropathy (see below).

Diabetic neuropathy. Among the many problems facing the diabetic is a painful neuropathy, which is caused by the nerve cells being starved of their favorite fuel: blood glucose. Diabetic neuropathy usually includes numbness, tingling and pain in the hands and feet. When diabetics were diligent about staying on their strict diet and following medication guidelines for blood glucose regulation, diabetic neuropathy was cut by 64%[11]. Other ways of controlling diabetic neuropathy include pain medication, of which the safest and most effective is cayenne ointment. Other analgesics (pain killers) that are widely used have numerous side effects. Kidney failure may accompany the excess use of Tylenol® and other drugs containing acetaminophen.

Axsain® is an ointment containing 0.075% capsaicin content. When applied topically, this ointment penetrates deeply into the skin to the surface nerves and depletes the nerves of substance P, which generates pain. Capsaicin ointments usually must be used for anywhere from 1-7 days before the pain killing effect is felt.

In one double blind study involving 227 men and women with painful diabetic neuropathy, 71% of capsaicin-treated patients reported improvement versus 51% in the placebo group[12]. Patients treated with the capsaicin ointment reported improvements in work, sleep, walking and participation in recreational activities. The capsaicin ointment was applied to the affected regions of the body 4 times daily and improvement was generally seen within a week. 63% of these patients reported the side effects of burning, stinging or warming sensation at the site of the ointment. But these side effects were minor and considered tolerable. Capsaicin depletes the substance P that causes pain, but still allows for normal pressure, heat and other sensations[13]. No medication can do what cayenne may be able to do for diabetics: knock out the pain yet still allow other sensations to the nerve endings without toxic side effects or addiction.

Fatigue & depression. As one of the most common symptoms reported to American physicians, fatigue and depression seem to be linked together. Cayenne, through some unknown mechanism, seems to excite and stimulate nerves[14]. The net effect is that many people feel energized by the regular use of capsaicin and hot chili peppers. The increased oxygen consumption of Thai people when eating hot chilis is similar to what is found with higher adrenaline output. Cayenne may be energizing people by stimulating the production of adrenaline, which definitely will relieve fatigue and possibly depression. A team of French scientists has found a definite energizing stimulating tonic effect from the consumption of hot chilis[15].

One of the more intriguing aspects of cayenne is the "high" experienced by the seasoned user of hot peppers. The body carries its own pharmacy in the brain. When we are hurt, burned or in shock, the brain sends out morphine-like compounds, called endorphins, to sooth the pain. Cayenne feels like it is burning the skin, but it doesn't. The brain sends out the required "medication" of endorphins to reduce the expected pain from this burn. Scientists have actually found receptor sites on human nerve cells for capsaicin[16]. You may find it equally puzzling that there are receptor sites in the human brain for caffeine (from coffee, tea, and colas), theophylline (from tea), alcohol (benzodiazepine sites in the brain), morphine and heroine (endorphin sites in the brain), nicotine (from tobacco), and THC from marijuana.

What scientists, like Dr. Candace Pert from the National Institutes of Health, are discovering is that the human brain is a pharmacy, always generating chemicals based upon your thoughts and state of health. These chemicals can be pleasurable or stressful. No doubt, there is a chemical produced in the human brain that is similar in active receptor site to capsaicin. By eating cayenne, we generate more of these healthful and pleasurable effects. In a similar fashion, exercise can cause the brain to release endorphins for pleasure.

Fatty liver. The liver is one of the largest and, arguably, the most sophisticated organ in the human body. It converts, stores, processes and detoxifies millions of molecules a minute. When the liver develops fatty accumulation, all of the vital functions in the liver slow down. Due to its lipotropic action (means "breaking up fats), cayenne may be able to help prevent the collection of fats in the liver. Cayenne may also reduce the toxic effects of alcohol, which can cause fatty liver, and possibly worse (fibrosis, necrosis).

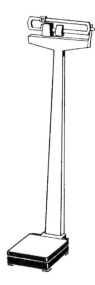

Fat reduction. Cayenne has the remarkable ability to favorably alter the levels of fats in the blood and the body. Country doctors have noticed for decades that people who eat lots of hot peppers rarely get overweight. In animals, giving capsaicin in the diet while feeding 30% of the calories as lard provided for a 29% reduction in serum triglycerides compared to animals fed the same diet but no capsaicin[17]. A human using cayenne pepper daily might expect to drop their triglycerides from 300 milligrams per deciliter, which puts them at risk for heart disease[18], to 213 mg per deciliter which is closer to the normal range. In the animal study just mentioned, there was a 24% reduction in fat surrounding the kidneys (perirenal). Through some unknown mechanism, cayenne helps the body to mobilize and use up fats, which is a very healthy effect for fat-burdened Americans. For more information, see "obesity" below.

Food poisoning. See "worms" below.

Frostbite. See "warming effect" below.

Gas (flatulence). While everyone from the President to the Pope does it, sometimes gas can become a troubling issue. Intestinal gas is more likely to be produced when we eat foods that we do not digest well, but putrefactive intestinal bacteria thrive on; such as beans and nuts. Cashews, peanuts, soybeans, and other beans can generate an embarrassing round of gas. Obviously, one solution is to reduce the intake of foods that generate gas.

Another strategy is to encourage the aerobic bacteria in the intestines which compete with the nasty putrefactive bacteria. Yogurt and capsules of Lactobacillus acidophilus (available at your health food store), and soil based organisms (from Nature's Biotics 810-629-9923 or online a www.natures-biotics.com) can help to generate a healthier climate in the human gut. More vegetables, less sugar and fat in the diet helps. Exercise helps to stimulate peristalsis, or the muscular movement of the intestines that pushes the food to its end point. When food is properly digested within a reasonable period of time, there is very little gas. When high fat food is allowed to ferment in the gut, there can be considerable gas.

Cayenne can reduce gas (a.k.a. carminative) in a number of ways:

1) As a stimulant, cayenne encourages the flow of secretions from the intestines, including digestive enzymes, which helps to prevent fermentation of carbohydrates in the gut

2) Cayenne moves food through the intestines more rapidly to reduce the chance of fermentation.

3) Cayenne helps to kill the unfriendly bacteria in the gut that cause gas through putrefaction, or literally turning your intestines into an old moonshiner's still.

The bottom line is that hot peppers and salsa will likely reduce the gas from your Mexican meal which usually includes gas-making beans.

Headache. Cluster headaches are common and can last up to 3 days for some unfortunate people. Medication for this condition usually centers around heavy narcotics which can make the patient drowsy. Cayenne may be the drug of choice for these people. Cluster headaches were treated by applying a topical capsaicin ointment to the inside of the sinuses. This should only be done under medical supervision. After 30 days of this treatment, 70% of the patients reported improvement in their cluster headaches[19]. In a separate study, 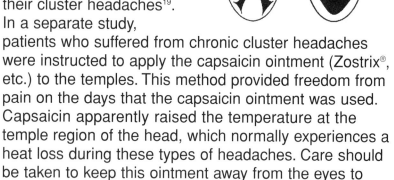 patients who suffered from chronic cluster headaches were instructed to apply the capsaicin ointment (Zostrix®, etc.) to the temples. This method provided freedom from pain on the days that the capsaicin ointment was used. Capsaicin apparently raised the temperature at the temple region of the head, which normally experiences a heat loss during these types of headaches. Care should be taken to keep this ointment away from the eyes to prevent stinging.

Heart disease. There are at least two famous medical herbalists, Dr. Richard Schulze[20] and Dr. John Ray Christopher who have written about their lifesaving experiences using cayenne to reverse congenital heart disease. For a particularly potent heart-protective herbal combination, use cayenne, garlic and hawthorne mixed together. See other sections under: fat reduction, high cholesterol, high blood pressure and obesity.

Heart arrhythmia. Irregular heart beat can be somewhere between annoying, frightening and life threatening, depending on how often it happens and for how long. Scientists using capsaicin to treat animals with heart arrhythmias found that capsaicin seemed to work like the prescription drugs, calcium channel blockers, to help regulate the heart beat[21].

Heat exhaustion. Not to be confused with heat stroke, which can be a fatal condition involving excess exposure to heat, with symptoms of headache, confusion, elevated skin temperature and eventually coma and death. For heat stroke, get medical help immediately. For heat exhaustion, which is characterized by weakness and general dehydration, cayenne, water and electrolytes can help.

For most of the 9000 years that hot peppers have been used, natives in warm climates noticed that chilis make the "dog days" of summer a little bit more bearable. The reason is that capsaicin causes peripheral vasodilation, or expansion of the blood vessels in the skin region[22]. When these blood vessels dilate and the inevitable sweating commences from eating hot chilis, the person is left with all of their natural cooling mechanisms in high gear. Sweating causes evaporation and a cooling effect. Dilating blood vessels in the skin brings the heat from the interior part of the body to the exterior for ventilation, not unlike the radiator on your car. In many different studies, scientists found that capsaicin generated a significant cooling effect[23]. You feel cooler and your body is better able to dissipate the heat buildup during those hot humid days. Drink plenty of pure water and eat hot chilis or take cayenne capsules throughout warm weather.

Herbal augmentor. With the stimulating and vasodilating effects of cayenne, cayenne is used along with other herbs to enhance their value. Hence, whether you are using saw palmetto for enlarged prostate or angelica for female fertility, cayenne improves the efficiency and delivery of nearly all herbal formulas.

High blood pressure (hypertension). About 50 million Americans suffer from hypertension. While there usually are no symptoms from this condition, it slowly wears out the vascular network and the organs connected. Hypertension is called the "silent killer", because the first symptom a person may have is a fatal stroke or heart attack. Cayenne may be able to help.

There is a heavily researched concept, called the calcitonin gene-related peptide or CGRP, which capsaicin can favorably influence to cause dilation of blood vessels. As mentioned above, capsaicin causes peripheral vasodilation, or expansion of the blood vessels in the skin region. High blood pressure can be caused by many factors, including stress, obesity, too much salt or alcohol, not enough calcium, magnesium, or potassium, not enough essential fatty acids and so on. When hypertension is caused by constriction of the blood vessels, which drives up the pressure in this narrower tubes, then cayenne can effectively reduce blood pressure in these people by expanding the diameter of the blood vessels. More room in the vessels means that the pressure goes down and you spare delicate capillaries in the kidney, liver, heart and brain region from the constant pounding of high blood pressure.

High cholesterol. With nearly one million Americans dying each year from heart disease and related disorders, cholesterol in the blood has become a valuable barometer of your overall health. When cholesterol "rusts" or oxidizes in the blood vessels, it creates free radical lipid peroxides that your immune cells gobble up to prevent any more damage from occurring. These immune cells then start stacking up dead in the blood vessel walls and are the beginning of vascular occlusions, which are found in 90% of Americans over age 30. Cholesterol is not as big a problem as "rusted" cholesterol, which is why other researchers have found that the level of vitamin E in the blood may be the most accurate indicator of upcoming heart disease, since vitamin E is the fat soluble antioxidant that protects the cholesterol from "rusting".

Capsaicin reduces the absorption of fats and cholesterol in the intestines, and slows down the making of excess cholesterol in the liver[24]. Whole cayenne powder was more effective at lowering serum fats than pure capsaicin[25], which is just another reason to rely heavily on the whole food more than some isolated extract (like capsaicin) as the only "active ingredient". In one study with animals, capsaicin in the diet was able to substantially drop serum cholesterol levels[26]. In another study with animals fed a high sugar and high fat diet (just like the typical American diet), capsaicin was able to lower the "bad" cholesterol (LDL and VLDL) and raise the "good" cholesterol (HDL[27]). As might be expected, countries that eat more hot peppers have a lower incidence of heart disease[28].

Libido, sex drive. Most Americans develop measurable "plugged up plumbing", or obstructed arteries, by the time they are in their 30s. In order for erections to occur, the penis must have clean and clear circulation in all the tiny capillaries that are supposed to become engorged with blood. In one study of 440 impotent men ages 40 and above, 92% had at least two major risk factors for heart disease, while 80% were found to have major blockage of the arteries[29], which means that the tiny capillaries in the penis region are likely also blocked. Another common reason for impotence is the use of hypertension medication, which causes a loss of potassium, magnesium and fluid from the body with the resulting inability to develop an erection.

Cayenne can help improve sex drive in several ways:

1) lower blood pressure, for some people to the point where you can discontinue medication

2) dilate and unblock blood vessels to allow the penis to be fully nourished and function as it should

3) stimulate and energize the nervous system.

Malnutrition. Hot chilis are rich in protein, fiber, complex carbohydrates, vitamins, minerals, bioflavonoids, carotenoids, and the magical capsaicin that has numerous benefits. Cayenne improves appetite and digestion. Thus hot peppers provide both direct nourishment and improvement in digestion and absorption of that nourishment. Altogether, hot peppers can help to prevent or reverse malnutrition when part of an overall balanced diet.

Mouth sores (oral mucositis). The incidence of cancer in this country has gone from 3% of deaths in 1900 to 23% of deaths in 2002 and climbing. More than 70% of cancer patients receive chemotherapy, which often causes mouth sores, a.k.a. oral mucositis. These painful blisters will stop the cancer patient from eating, which generates severe malnutrition and a compromised immune system. Mouth sores can be the beginning of the end for the cancer patient.

At the Yale Pain Management Center in New Haven, Connecticut, researchers devised an ingenious method of delivering capsaicin to cancer patients with mouth sores. The researchers mixed the cayenne with taffy candy. As reported in the prestigious *Journal of the National Cancer Institute,* the sugar was able to hide some of the burning sensation and the taffy stayed in the mouth long enough for the capsaicin to do its topical pain control management. All of the 11 patients in the study had significant decrease in mouth sore pain, with 2 patients reporting complete elimination of pain[30]. To follow this protocol, mix up some taffy from your favorite recipe book and add several capsules of cayenne powder to the mix.

Nausea. Take a teaspoon of cayenne powder mixed in a tablespoon of olive oil before beginning a trip where motion sickness may be a problem. Other herbalists[31] recommend an equal blend of ginger, cayenne, and licorice to prevent and relieve motion sickness and other forms of nausea. For morning sickness in pregnancy, use just the ginger and cayenne mixture.

Neuralgia. This is a pain of a severe throbbing or stabbing nature and can be found anywhere in the body. For relief, see the section "Pain".

Obesity. Although Americans have been in the midst of a "fitness revolution" and rivers of diet soft drinks have been consumed since the FDA approval of aspartame (NutraSweet®) in 1982, we now have a 30% increase in the incidence of obesity. Overweight people are more likely to die young of heart disease, diabetes, or various cancers, especially of the breast and colon. Cayenne can help.

There is a region of fatty tissue, called "brown adipose tissue" or BAT, found on the back and buttocks region of people. BAT is so named because it is much more loaded with blood vessels than regular white fatty storage regions. BAT is our body's thermogenic regulator, our internal "wood burning stove", which is supposed to squander excess stored fat in the making of heat. In many people, due to inactivity, wearing too much clothes, keeping the home thermostat set too high and exposure to psychological stress; we end up letting the BAT atrophy. Under ideal conditions, BAT takes excess fat in the body and burns it to maintain the ideal body temperature of 98.6 F. When BAT atrophies, it becomes very difficult for many people to lose weight. Ephedra from the Chinese herb, Ma Huang, along with white willow bark (aspirin) and Gotu Kola (caffeine) have been shown to stimulate BAT into action to help people lose weight. Cayenne also stimulates BAT[32]. One of the simplest things anyone can do to slowly and safely lose weight is to eat cayenne and other hot peppers to gear up the burning of stored fats in BAT. This simple procedure requires no change in diet and no exercise. It just increases the amount of calories being burned while at rest. Of course, if you do exercise and eat a low fat diet, the weight will melt away much quicker.

Osteoarthritis. Cartilage tissue normally cushions the connections between the bones. When this cartilage deteriorates, osteoarthritis is the result. This condition is actually bone rubbing against bone, which is painful and can immobilize people. Nearly 21 million Americans, mostly over age 45, are affected by osteoarthritis[33]. The drug of choice for osteoarthritis for many years has been NSAIDs, or non-steroidal anti-inflammatory drugs, like Advil®. NSAIDs come with a long grocery list of complications and side effects, including stomach upset, ulceration of the small intestine and colon, kidney failure, liver failure, skin reactions and interfering with high blood pressure medication[34]. Other prescription drugs sometimes used for osteoarthritis include morphine or codeine and steroid hormones, all of which have a lengthy list of complications, including addiction.

Cayenne to the rescue. Capsaicin ointments are sometimes referred to as "rubefacients", since they are counter-irritants which initially cause reddening on the skin. Be aware that many capsaicin "rubefacient" ointments also contain nicotine (methyl niconate) and aspirin (methyl salicylate) in small enough quantities to be of little concern. However, capsaicin ointment alone (no other therapy, no other ingredients in the ointment) was able to provide significant relief of osteoarthritis pain in a 12 week double blind study[35].

Pain. Here we find one of the many paradoxes regarding cayenne. It seems to cause pain when you eat it or rub it on the skin. Yet, it actually reduces pain by depleting the nerve endings of Substance P (for pain)[36]. Researchers also find that capsaicin has some mysterious effect on calcium levels in the nerve endings[37]. Up to 20% of the adult population (50 million Americans) suffer from chronic pain, while half of them are inadequately treated[38].

Cayenne ointment has been clinically proven to help relieve the pain of:

⇒ shingles (herpes zoster, or postherpetic neuralgia)
⇒ skin diseases
⇒ psoriasis (red scaly lesions on the skin)
⇒ pruritus (itching)
⇒ peripheral neuropathy
⇒ fibromyalgia, which is an arthritis-like condition from Chronic Fatigue Syndrome[39].
⇒ post-mastectomy pain
⇒ stump pain from amputation
⇒ trigeminal neuralgia
⇒ skin cancer

Axsain®, Arthri-Gel® (GeroVita International 800-406-1314) and Zostrix® are capsaicin ointments that are available over-the-counter. Pain relief usually begins after several days of using these ointments.

Researchers have discovered a "mother lode" of healing possibilities in nitric oxide, a substance found throughout the body regulating everything from nerve conduction to the immune system. Capsaicin apparently affects nitric oxide levels.

Patients who undergo a mastectomy for breast cancer often suffer with pain in the surgical region.

Capsaicin creme applied 3 times daily for 2 months produced improvements in post-mastectomy pain syndrome in 68% of the patients[40].

There is a condition called trigeminal neuralgia, which involves a stabbing pain in the facial region. Topical capsaicin used three times daily provided complete relief of the pain in half (6 of 12) of the subjects and partial relief in a third (4 of 12) of the subjects for an 83% response rate with no addictions, side effects or long term toxicities[41].

When Substance P is allowed to run amuck, for those willing to tolerate the pain, it can eventually contribute to erosion of the joint endings and result in osteoarthritis. Chronic pain is not something to be endured, since it can lead to even more disabling joint conditions. Capsaicin ointment has become the "drug of choice" to treat many forms of pain, including peripheral neuropathy (tingling numbness in the extremities), local stump pain (from amputation), hyperalgesia (extreme sensitivity to pain response), pain from skin cancer and more.

Parasites. See "worms" below.

Pesticide. Foxes in the Arctic started chewing through important scientific cables. The researchers found that spreading cayenne powder over slightly tacky silicone sealant that was applied to the cables was able to stop the foraging foxes from this costly habit. Other gardeners have found that cayenne can keep out many rabbits, raccoons, deer, insects and other pests. However, birds seem unaffected by the pungency of cayenne. Other animals have developed a penchant for cayenne. Cayenne is an inexpensive and non-toxic pesticide, but I wouldn't "bet the farm on it" as a universal pesticide agent.

Pleurisy. This condition involves the inflammation of the lining of the lungs. Cayenne is a stimulant and vasodilator that may help this condition. Do not inhale cayenne powder, but rather take 2 capsules of cayenne powder (40,000 heat units or higher) with lunch and dinner.

You can also use a time-tested herbalist's favorite rub for speeding the relief of pleurisy. Mix equal parts of powdered cayenne pepper, lobelia herb and slippery elm bark into a small amount of cod liver oil (all found at your health food store). Use just enough cod liver oil to form a thick paste like Vaseline® jelly. Apply this paste to the affected region of the chest every 3 hours, then cover with plastic wrap, then a clean flannel cloth. Be sure to wash your hands afterwards.

Psoriasis. Psoriasis is a common, painful and embarrassing skin condition involving red scaly formations throughout the body, usually centered on the elbows, knees and arms. Several studies have shown the impressive results from using capsaicin ointment in psoriasis. In one study, 44 patients with widely distributed psoriasis used a capsaicin ointment on one side of the body and a placebo ointment on the other side of the body. After six weeks, there was considerable improvement in scaling and redness (erythema) on the sides of the body treated with capsaicin[42]. In another much larger study, 197 patients with itching psoriasis were treated in double blind fashion with half of the patients randomly assigned to getting capsaicin ointment and the other half of the patients getting a placebo ointment. The psoriasis was totally or markedly cleared in 82% of the capsaicin treated group versus 33% in the placebo group[43].

Shingles (herpes zoster). Many children suffer through chicken pox, which is provided to us compliments of the herpes zoster virus. This virus may then lay dormant in the body for decades and re-surface in senior years when the immune system is compromised by poor diet, stress or whatever. The new batch of herpes zoster is often called shingles, and is an extremely painful condition, since the virus attacks the nerves in the skin region. In 7 studies using capsaicin ointment to treat the pain of shingles, ALL showed a substantial decrease in the pain score[44]. In one study, doctors instructed patients suffering from shingles pain (post herpetic neuralgia) to apply capsaicin ointment 4 times a day to the affected painful area. After 8 weeks, 49% of the patients reported improvements in pain, but 13% discontinued the use of the creme due to the burning sensation. Relief was usually noticed within the first 3 weeks and pain relief peaked at 5 weeks[45].

Sinusitis. One of the more frequent complaints among Americans is sinus problems. This problem is often generated by the common allergies from milk, wheat, ragweed, pollen and the irritation of air pollution. Many Americans develop sinus congestion or continuous sinus flow. Rhinitis is an inflammation of the nasal mucus membranes, which is related to sinusitis and also very common. Cayenne may be able to help. Researchers found that "painting" a capsaicin solution on the nasal membranes in the nose eventually was able to cure chronic rhinitis[46]. This medically supervised procedure may be uncomfortable, but it may also be worth the effort. As an alternative to painting your sinus regions with capsaicin ointment, try taking 2 capsules of cayenne powder with lunch and dinner.

A favorite herbalist's remedy for sinusitis is to mix 1/4 teaspoon each of cayenne powder and garlic powder in with a bowl of hot chicken soup. Drink it down with gusto. Usually relieves the stuffy nose and sneezing.

Skin problems. Since cayenne is such a potent stimulant and vasodilator, it can be very helpful in clearing up minor skin problems, from acne to psoriasis to dry skin. Take 2 capsules of 40,000+ heat unit cayenne with lunch and dinner. Try applying one of the previously mentioned capsaicin ointments on the affected skin region. For the bold readers, mix 1 capsule of cayenne powder with a small amount of pure aloe vera gel. Apply to acne or dry skin at night. Make sure that you do not get any of this solution into your eyes. Wash hands after applying to face. See section for "psoriasis".

Sore throat. With the stimulating effects of cayenne, it has been found to be a valuable component to reduce the severity and duration of sore throats. Mix 1-2 capsules of cayenne powder (40,000 heat units or higher) in 1 cup of warm water. Swish in your mouth and gargle, but do not swallow. If this preparation is too hot to tolerate, then cut the cayenne in half and try again.

Stress reducer. Animals given cayenne have been found to better tolerate physical and psychological stress. Cayenne is a stimulant and encourages the transmission of nerve impulses, therefore it will offer better stress tolerance in regular users.

Stroke. Your body has 60,000 miles of blood vessels which create a complete network of circulation to each and every cell in the human body. In many Americans, due to stress, high fat diet, wrong kind of fat in the diet, sedentary lifestyle, and low intake of vitamin E and fish oil--our blood turns from a thin liquid into a thick sludgy liquid that is unable to feed the distant tissues in the body. This thicker blood is constantly forming clots, or embolisms, in various parts of the body. When these clots form in the brain, a stroke can be the result. Over 163,000 Americans died last year from strokes, or cerebrovascular problems. Those who do survive a stroke often end up with partial paralysis, or a loss of speech or memory. Cayenne to the rescue.

Hot peppers thin the blood by breaking up these clots. People who eat lots of hot chilis have a very low incidence of blood clots (thromboembolism[47]). The people in Thailand, who are world renowned chiliheads, have a full 33% reduction in the clotting tendency of their blood when compared to the typical American. This beneficial effect from cayenne serves many purposes. Obviously, it cuts the risk for stroke or embolism. But more importantly, and not as obviously, cayenne thins the blood to help this "river of life" to circulate throughout the body to feed the distant tissues.

In one study, a scientist placed a sample of chicken heart tissue in a Petri dish full of nutrient solution. Everyday he changed the solution to take away waste products and renew the nutrient supply surrounding this tissue. The tissue basically never aged. When we bring in the right amount of groceries and take out the trash (detoxify the cells), we seem to slow down the aging process and improve our vitality. Cayenne does this and more.

Thyroid problems. Do you suffer from any of the following symptoms: constipation, fatigue, depression, poorly regulated or painful menstrual cycles, hair loss, easy weight gain, allergies, heart disease, and poor tolerance to cold temperatures? If so, then you may have an easily corrected problem: hypothyroidism. According to a huge amount of scientific literature on this subject, up to 40% of the American public suffers from mild to severe hypothyroidism. Stephen Langer, MD[48]; Denis Wilson, MD[49] and Broda Barnes, MD, PhD[50] have been pioneers in alerting the public to this fundamental health problem. If your basal temperature first thing in the morning is below 97.8 F, then you may have hypothy- roidism. This simple and easily corrected issue may make a huge difference in your overall health.

Cayenne may be able to help. Herbalists find that a mixture of cayenne (since it is a potent stimulant) along with kelp, gentian root, and Irish moss may be able to stimulate the thyroid back into full action. Otherwise, it may be necessary to find a physician willing to recommend prescription thyroid supplements to gear up the lagging thyroid gland.

Toothache. The earliest report in the medical literature for therapeutic uses of hot peppers comes from an 1850 report in an Irish medical journal which used 1-2 drops of hot pepper extract applied to a cotton swab and then to the toothache gum region[51]. Since capsaicin is easily dissolved in alcohol, one way to make this toothache tincture is to blend 2 capsules of 40,000 heat unit cayenne powder in 4 ounces of gin. Let sit for a day. Strain. Apply a few drops of this tincture to the toothache region.

Toxin protection. Cayenne helps to encourage sweating. The skin is the largest organ in the human body, with about 2000 pores per square inch of surface area. A main function of the skin is to eliminate waste products. You may recall a James Bond film called GoldFinger, in which a young secretary was sprayed completely over with gold paint - and died from having her pores closed up and unable to breathe. Cayenne encourages sweating and detoxification, which is an extremely important function in toxically burdened Americans[52].

Ulcers. While it may seem odd that cayenne can actually help to heal a stomach ulcer, scientific evidence points us in that direction. People in Malaysia and India eat much more hot peppers and have fewer stomach ulcers than people in China. Studies since 1937 have shown that people who eat more hot peppers get fewer stomach problems, including ulcers[53]. And while no one will argue that TOO MUCH hot peppers will produce stomach irritation and eventually ulcers, just the right amount will prevent and even cure ulcers. Scientists find that capsaicin may help heal ulcers by:
⇨ dilating blood vessels in the stomach region, which accelerates healing
⇨ increasing the flow of protective mucus over the ulcer

⇒ killing the bacteria, Helicobacter pylori, which causes many cases of peptic ulcer.

Dr. D.Y. Graham and colleagues reported in the *Journal of the American Medical Association* that administering a healthy dose (30 grams or one ounce) of jalapeño alone in the stomach did not cause any gastric erosion based upon their endoscope exams. Yet these researchers did find that taking aspirin with a bland meal caused measurable gastric erosion (the makings of an ulcer) in 11 out of 12 subjects[54].

One of the most common causes of ulcers in America is the excessive use of aspirin, which provokes microscopic bleeding in the stomach wall. When researchers gave volunteers 20 grams of chilis (less than an ounce) 30 minutes before giving 600 milligrams of aspirin (a routine dose), the damage from the aspirin was substantially reduced[55].

Another common cause of ulcers in America is alcohol consumption, which irritates the stomach lining. In animal studies, a reasonable amount of chili intake was able to protect the stomach from damage by alcohol, even when the animals were fasted for 24 hours before alcohol was given[56]. If you do drink alcohol, then cayenne may help reduce the damage to the stomach from alcohol.

Urinary tract pain. Medical administration of capsaicin to the bladder has been very effective in reducing pain[57]. Capsaicin supplements taken orally have been helpful in reducing the pain in urination and frequency of urination (micturition[58]). Take 1-2 capsules of cayenne powder with lunch and dinner.

Warming effect. Since cayenne is such a potent vasodilator, it has been used to help speed the sensation of feeling in frostbitten hands and feet. The Denver Broncos professional football team used cayenne rubbed on the feet to keep their feet warm while playing in a blizzard in December of 1987 against the San Diego Chargers[59]. The Broncos won the game. In order to try this, for you snowmobilers out there, sprinkle cayenne pepper in your socks. Or, liquify a small container of petroleum jelly in the microwave, then mix in 3-4 capsules of cayenne powder and let cool before applying to skin. Remember, your feet may "feel" hot, but you may be losing body heat at a faster rate, so watch the possibilities of frostbite.

Worms. Ask any farmer, or veterinarian or pet owner about the need to purge worms and parasites from the colon of ALL animals. Medication, called a vermifuge or anthelmintic, is given often to animals to clean out the inevitable worms and parasites that collect in the digestive tract. These worms and parasites sap us of energy, change the environment in the gut and lower the immune system. Although the sanitation at our dinner table is, no doubt, much better than a dog's dinner bowl or a cow's feeding trough, many humans are afflicted with parasites and worms[60].

Cayenne can help. At a meeting for the American Society for Microbiology held at Louisiana State University, scientists reported the extraordinary ability of hot sauce to kill microorganisms, including a bacteria (Vibrio vulnificus) that is commonly found in oysters and can cause serious health problems in humans eating the oysters. Hot sauce killed the more common intestinal infections (shigella, E. coli, and salmonella) in one minute flat. Ever notice how "gringos" seem vulnerable to the tap water in many Latin American countries? Maybe all that hot sauce in the local's diet is a major protector against worms, parasites and bacterial food poisoning. Next time someone warns you "don't drink the water", reach for some extra cayenne for that meal.

ENDNOTES

[1]. American Herart Assn; Heart Disease and Stroke Statistical Update, 2004
[2]. Rubino, A., et al., Cardiovascular Research, vol.31, p.467, 1996
[3]. Cerinic, MM, et al., Journal of Rheumatology, vol.22, no.8, p.1447, 1995
[4]. McCarthy, GM, et al., Journal Rheumatology, vol.19, p.604, 1992
[5]. Colpaert, FC, et al., Life Sciences, vol.32, p.1827, 1983
[6]. Lopez-Carillo, L., et al., American Journal Epidemiology, vol.139, p.263, 1994
[7]. Surh, YJ, et al., Food Chemical Toxicology, vol.34, p.313, 1996
[8]. Unnikrishnan, MC, et al., Cancer Letters, vol.51, p.85, 1990
[9]. Dib, B, Pharmacol Biochem Behav., vol.28, p.65, 1987
[10]. Monsereenusorn, Y., Q.J.Crude Drug Research, vol.18, p.1, 1980
[11]. Emanuele, NV, et al., Comprehensive Therapy, vol.21, no.10, p.579, 1995
[12]. Diabetes Care, vol.15, p.159, 1992
[13]. Tandan, R., et al., Diabetes Care, vol.15, no.1, p.8, 1992
[14]. O'Neil, TP, Respiratory Medicine, vol.85, suppl.A, p.35, 1991
[15]. Roquebert, J., et al., Annales Pharmaceutiques Francaises, vol.36, p.361, 1978
[16]. Bevan, S., et al., British Journal of Pharmacology, p.32, May 1991
[17]. Kawada, T., et al., Journal Nutrition, vol.116, p.1272, 1986
[18]. Wallach, J., INTERPRETATION OF DIAGNOSTIC TESTS, p.465, Little, Brown, Boston, 1996
[19]. Fusco, BM, et al., Pain, vol.59, p.321, 1994
[20]. Biser, S., CURING WITH CAYENNE, Univ.Natural Healing, Charlottesville, VA, 1997
[21]. D'Alonzo, AJ, et al., European Journal Pharmacology, vol.272, p.269, Jan.1995
[22]. Bell, D., et al., Pharmacological Reviews, vol.48, no.2, p.253, 1996
[23]. Govindarajan, VS, et al., Critical Reviews in Food Science & Nutrition, vol.29, no.6, p.435, 1991
[24]. Sambaiah, K., et al., Nutrition Reports International, vol.18, p.521, 1978
[25]. Srinivasan, MR, et al., Nutrition Reports International, vol.21, p.455, 1980
[26]. Ki, P, et al., IRCS Medical Science Library Compendium, vol.10, p.446, 1982
[27]. Srinivasan, MR, et al., Nutrition Reports International, vol.38, no.3, p.571, 1988
[28]. Ki, P, et al., IRCS Medical Science Biochemistry, vol.10, p.446, 1982
[29]. Virag, R., et al., Lancet, p.183, Jan.26, 1985
[30]. Nelson, C., Journal National Cancer Institute, vol.86, p. 1381, 1994
[31]. Mowrey, DB, SCIENTIFIC VALIDATION OF HERBAL MEDICINE, p.197, Keats, New Canaan, CT, 1986
[32]. Yoshida, T., Journal Nutrition Science Vitaminology, vol.34, p.587, 1988
[33]. Arthristis Foundation, Osteoartritis, 2003

34. Berkow, R. (ed), MERCK MANUAL, p.1232, 16th ed.Merck, Rahway, NJ 1992
35. Altman, RD, et al., Arthritis Rheumatology, vol.23, suppl.3, p.25, 1994
36. Bernstein, JE, Clinics in Dermatology, vol.9, p.497, 1992
37. Winter, J., et al., British Journal Anaesthesia, vol.75, p.157, 1995
38. Perkins, M., et al., Annals Rheumatic Diseases, vol.55, p.715, 1996
39. Markovits, E., International Journal Dermatology, vol.36, p.401, 1997
40. Dini, D, et al., Pain, vol.54, p.223, 1993
41. Fusco, BM, et al., Anesthesia Analgesics, vol.74, p.375, 1992
42. Bernstein, JE, et al., Journal American Academy Dermatology, vol.15, p.504, 1986
43. Breberian, B., et al., Journal Investigative Dermatology, vol.94, p.506, 1990
44. Palevitch, D., et al., Journal of Herbs, Spices & Medicinal Plants, vol.3, no.2, p.55, 1995
45. Peikert, A., et al., Journal Neurology, vol.238, p.452, 1991
46. Lacroix, JS, et al., Clinical Experience Allergy, vol.21, p.595, 1991
47. Visudhiphan, S., et al., American Journal Clinical Nutrition, vol.35, p.1452, 1982
48. Langer, SE, SOLVED THE RIDDLE OF ILLNESS, Keats, New Canaan, CT, 1984
49. Wilson, ED, WILSON'S SYNDROME, Cornerstone, Orlando, 1991
50. Barnes, BO, et al., HYPOTHYROIDISM, Harper & Row, NY, 1976
51. Turnbull, A., Dublin Medical Press, vol.1, p.95, 1850
52. Lee, TS, Journal of Physiology, vol.124, p.528, 1954
53. Kang, JY, Singapore Medical Journal, vol.33, p.468, 1992
54. Graham, DY, et al., Journal American Medical Association, vol.260, p.3473, 1988
55. Yeoh, KG, et al., Digestive Disease Science, vol.40, p.580, 1995
56. Kang, JY, et al., Gut, vol.36, p.664, 1995
57. Barbanti, G, et al., British Journal Urology, vol.71, p.686, 1993
58. Maggi, CA, et al., Journal Urology, vol.142, p.150, 1989
59. DeWitt, D., et al., HEAT WAVE, p.131, Crossing Press, Freedom, CA, 1995
60. Gittleman, AL, GUESS WHAT CAME TO DINNER, Avery, Garden City Park, NY, 1993

Chapter Three

Cooking with Hot Chilis

by Noreen Quillin & Patrick Quillin

While using cayenne as a capsule or powder on your food is an effective way of gaining the health benefits, you may want to sample some of the following recipes to see if you can also benefit from the flavor of hot peppers.

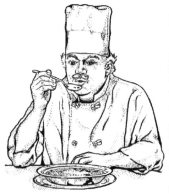

How to peel fresh green chilis. Wash and wipe dry. Arrange peppers close together in a broiler pan; place 1 inch from the heat in a preheated broiler. Turn chilis often until they are blistered and lightly browned all over. As the chilis are done, drop them into a paper bag; then close the bag. When cool enough to handle, peel off loose skin with a knife; leave any small pieces that refuse to come off easily. For a milder flavor; cut the chili open and remove the seeds.

USING CHILIS AS SEASONINGS

Chili Water
2 jalapeño chilis
2 Tbs. minced ginger
2 Tbs. vinegar
1 clove garlic
1/8 tsp. sea salt
2 cups water
Remove the stems and seeds from the chilis. Puree in a blender; the chilis, ginger, vinegar, garlic, salt and 1/2 cup of water. Bring the rest of the water to a boil and add the puree. Bring the mixture to a boil. Remove from the stove and place in a glass jar. Keep it in the refrigerator after it has cooled. Use a few tablespoons as a soup base and in cooking.

Soup or Salad Seasoning
1 tsp. ground chili
2 tsp. onion powder
1 tsp. ground allspice
1 tsp. ground thyme
2 tsp. ground cinnamon
1 tsp. ground cloves
1/4 tsp. ground nutmeg
1/4 tsp. ground mace
1/2 tsp. garlic powder
1/2 tsp. pepper
1/2 tsp. salt
Mix the ingredients together and use in a salt shaker. Use liberally to spice up your food.

Creole Seasoning

12 oz. salt
1/2 oz. black pepper
1 oz. cayenne pepper
1/2 oz. garlic powder
1/2 oz. chili powder

Blend ingredients and store in a jar with a tight lid. Makes about one and a half cups of seasoning.

Creole Seafood Seasoning

1/6 cup salt
1/6 cup paprika
1/8 cup black pepper
1/8 cup garlic powder
1 1/2 Tbs. onion powder
1 Tbs. cayenne pepper
1 Tbs. oregano
1 Tbs. thyme

Combine all ingredients and mix. Keeps indefinitely in a tightly sealed glass jar. Makes one cup.

Roasted Nut Meal

1 cup toasted nuts of your choice or combination
1/4 cup toasted sesame or sunflower seeds
1 1/4 tsp. chili powder
1/2 tsp. cumin powder
1/8 tsp. garlic powder
1/8 tsp. onion powder
1/8 tsp. clove powder
2 Tbs. nutritional yeast (opt.)

Blend all ingredients in blender until nuts make a nut meal. Use to sprinkle on grains, vegetables, or salad dishes.

COOKING WITH HOT CHILIS

Hot Bean Paste
6 dried red chilis
1 can (15-16 oz.) red beans
1/2 cup water
1/2 tsp. cornstarch
1 tsp. vinegar
3 cloves garlic, chopped
2 Tbs. onion, minced fine
1 Tbs. vegetable oil
1/4 tsp. salt

Remove stems and seeds from the chilis. Place the chilis in hot water for 15 minutes or until soft. Drain and chop. Strain the beans and puree in a blender until smooth. Use some of the bean liquid if necessary. Mix 1 tablespoon of the water with the cornstarch and vinegar.

Saute the chilis, garlic and onion in the oil. Add the beans, salt and the rest of the water. Cover and simmer for 20 minutes. Stir in the cornstarch and simmer for 12 minutes more. Refrigerate in a glass jar.

USING CHILIS IN SAUCES

Apple Chutney
5 lbs. apples
1/2 cup water
1/4 cup butter
1/2 tsp. crushed chili pepper
1 Tbs. canned California diced green chilis
1 tsp. nutmeg
1/2 tsp. allspice
1 tsp. ginger
1 1/2 tsp. cinnamon
dash nutmeg
1 1/2 cups honey

Peel, core, and chop apples into quarters. Steam apples in water until tender. When done, remove lid and cook off excess water, being careful not to burn. In a deep skillet , heat butter and toast spices. Add apples and chilis. Cook away excess liquid on high heat, stirring often. Add honey and cook on medium heat until jamlike, stirring frequently to prevent sticking and burning. Remove from heat, allow to cool, then refrigerate. Can be served warm, but it is better chilled.

Garlic chili
6 dried red New Mexican chilis
1 1/4 tsp. garlic powder
1/8 tsp. onion powder

Remove the stems and seeds from the chilis and cover with water. Boil for 15 minutes. Puree all ingredients together in a blender until smooth. Allow to cool before serving.

Seafood Salsa
2 Habañero chilis
2 limes, juiced
2 Tbs. water
1/8 tsp. garlic powder
1/3 head cabbage, grated
1 onion, finely chopped
     Remove stems and seeds from chilis. Mince chilis. Mix the lime juice and water. Pour over rest of the ingredients in a bowl. Mix.

Easy Salsa
5-6 Jalapeño chilis
1 large onion, minced
2 medium tomatoes, minced
1 Tbs. cilantro, minced
2 Tbs. parsley, minced
1/4 cup red wine vinegar
1/4 cup olive oil
     Remove stems and seeds from chilis. Mince fine. Mix all the ingredients together. Cover and leave at room temperature for about an hour.

Serrano Salsa
5 Serrano chilis
1/2 pound tomatillos, chopped
1/2 cup onion, minced
1 Tbs. cilantro, minced
1 Tbs. parsley, minced
1/4 tsp. salt
     Remove stems and seeds from chilis. Chop. Place all ingredients in a blender and puree. You might need to add a bit of water. You want the sauce to be thick.

Seafood Taco Salsa

5 dried Habañero chilis, stems remove
1/4 cup onion, chopped
1 pound mangos, peeled and chopped
2 Tbs. golden raisins
1/8 tsp. ground turmeric
1 fresh lime, juiced

     Cover the chilis with water in a saucepan. Add onions. Simmer until chilis are soft. Add the mango and raisins and bring to the beginning of a boil. Remove from heat. Place all the ingredients in a blender and puree.

Peach Salsa

3 large peaches
1/3 cup fructose
2/3 cup peach juice
2 Tbs. vinegar
3 Tbs. dried red New Mexican chili, crushed
1/4 tsp. cinnamon
1/4 tsp. ground cumin

     Peel and dice the peaches. Dissolve the fructose in the peach juice and vinegar. Add the chili, cinnamon, and cumin. Bring to a boil, then simmer for 20 minutes. Add the peaches and simmer for 5 minutes. This is great with grilled food.

Relish Salsa

6 cloves garlic, minced
1/4 cup lemon juice
1 1/2 Tbs. olive oil
1 1/2 Tbs. parsley, minced
1 tsp. crushed New Mexican red chili
salt and pepper to taste

Mix the ingredients and place in a nonreactive container. Refrigerate overnight. Let the mixture sit at room temperature for about an hour before serving.

Avocado Chili
1/4 cup Serrano chilis
1/4 cup Jalapeño chilis
1/4 cup onion, chopped
1/2 cup lime juice
1/4 tsp. sea salt
3 tomatoes, chopped fine, keep juice
1/4 cup parsley, minced
1 large avocado, chopped fine
        Place the first 5 ingredients in a nonreactive bowl. Mix. Refrigerate for 1 hour. Drain off the lime juice. Add the rest of the ingredients. Serve.

Green Chili Sauce
12 green chilis, finely chopped
2 tomatoes, finely chopped
2-3 cloves garlic, minced
1 onion, diced
salt, optional
        Place all the ingredients in a saucepan. Add enough water to just cover. Simmer over medium low heat for 10 minutes. Add salt to taste.

Chili Wine Sauce
6 green chilis, roasted and peeled
1 onion, minced
3 cloves garlic, minced
1 Tbs. canola oil
1 Tbs. whole wheat flour
1 tomato, chopped
1 cup water

2/3 cup white wine (or water)
    Chop the chilis. Saute the onion and garlic in the oil. Add the flour. Toast the flour lightly. Add all of the ingredients and bring to a boil. Reduce the heat and simmer for 30 minutes.

Hot Hot Chili Sauce
12 chili de arbols
2 1/2 Tbs. apple cider vinegar
3 cloves garlic
1/2 tsp. dried oregano
1/2 tsp. salt
1/2 tsp. dry parsley
1/4 tsp. ground cumin
1/2 tsp. salt
1/2 cup water

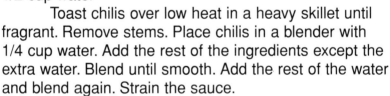

    Toast chilis over low heat in a heavy skillet until fragrant. Remove stems. Place chilis in a blender with 1/4 cup water. Add the rest of the ingredients except the extra water. Blend until smooth. Add the rest of the water and blend again. Strain the sauce.

Enchilada Sauce
10 dried New Mexican chilis
1 large onion, chopped
4 cloves garlic, chopped
1 Tbs. canola oil
1 Tbs. dried parsley
2 2/3 cups water
1/2 tsp. dried oregano
    Bake chilis on a baking pan in a preheated 240 degree oven for about 10 minutes until chilis smell like they are toasted.

Saute the onion and garlic in the oil in a sauce pan until soft. Remove stems and seeds from the chilis and crumble into the sauce pan. Add the rest of the ingredients and simmer for 25 minutes. Puree in a blender until smooth. Strain.

USING CHILIS IN APPETIZERS

Spicy Peanuts
10 small dried red chilis
3 cloves garlic, minced fine
1/2 Tbs. olive oil
1 pound salted peanuts
1/2 tsp. chili powder

Fry chilis, garlic and oil for 1 minute. Stir the full minute. Mix in the nuts and fry until lightly brown. Sprinkle on the chili powder. Mix well. Cool. Make this snack up the day before.

Chili Cheese Dip
6 fresh California green chilis
1/2 Tbs. canola oil
1 onion, chopped
1 clove garlic, minced fine
1/2 tsp. salt
2 1/2 oz. evaporated milk
pinch cumin (opt.)
2/3 cup shredded cheddar cheese
Baked corn chips

Wash and dry the chilis. Peel the chilis as directed in the beginning of this section. Remove seeds if you want it more mild. Chop the chilis.

Saute onions and garlic in the oil. Add the chilis and salt and cook for about 5 minutes. Add the evaporated milk and optional cumin and cook gently for 4 minutes.

Remove from heat. After one minute, add cheese and cover. Stir after the cheese melts. Serve hot with chips.

Stuffed Hot Chilis
1/2 pound lean ground beef
1 onion, diced
2 cloves garlic, crushed
1/4 cup raisins
10 black olives, sliced
1 cup cooked brown rice, measured after cooking
2 ounces grated gouda cheese
12 large yellow chilis

 Brown the beef, onion and garlic. Remove from heat. Add the rest of the ingredients. Cut stems out of each chili and remove the seeds. Keep the top. Stuff the chilis with the mixture. Seal the hole with the top of the chili. Bake in a preheated 350 degree oven, covered, for 20 minutes.

Stuffed Mushrooms
8 large mushrooms
1 Tbs. butter
1 spring onion, finely chopped
1 clove garlic, minced
1 Tbs. parsley, finely chopped
1 tsp. chili powder
1/4 cup dry whole wheat cracker crumbs
1/4 cup feta cheese, crumbled fine

 Twist the stems off the mushrooms. Finely chop the stems. Saute the onion, stems and garlic in the butter. Remove from heat. Add the rest of the ingredients. Mix well. Stuff the mushrooms with the filling. Make a mound of the filling. Place mushrooms, filling side up, in a baking dish sprayed with vegetable oil. Bake in a preheated 350 degree oven for 20 minutes.

Raw Fish Appetizer
1 1/2 pounds sole (or other mild-flavored fish)
1 cup lemon juice
2 canned California green chilis, seeded and chopped
1/2 cup onion, minced
1 clove garlic, minced (opt.)
2 tomatoes, chopped
1 tsp. salt
1/4 tsp. oregano leaves, crushed
1 tsp. dry parsley, crushed
1/4 cup olive oil

Cut fish in small, thin slices. Place in a bowl with the lemon juice and refrigerate for 2 hours. Stir in the rest of the ingredients. Serve in chilled cups.

USING CHILIS IN SOUPS AND SALADS

Yogurt Dressing
1 can (4 oz.) diced California green chilis
1 cup plain yogurt
2 Tbs. minced onion
1 tsp. Dijon mustard
1/4 tsp. garlic salt
pepper
 Mix all of the ingredients and refrigerate for at least an hour.

Gazpacho
2 medium tomatoes, chopped
1 small onion, diced
1/2 cucumber, peeled
and diced
1/2 avocado, chopped
2 Tbs. canned mild green
diced chilis
1/2 tsp. oregano leaves,
crumbled
1/2 Tbs. parsley, chopped
2 Tbs. wine vinegar
2 Tbs. olive oil
4 cups canned tomato
juice
2 limes

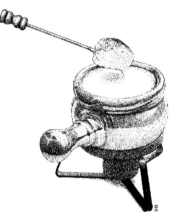

 Put the first 9 ingredients into a serving bowl. Stir in the tomato juice. Chill. Serve with lime juice to taste.

Black Bean Soup
2 cups dried black beans
2 quarts water
8 cups chicken broth
1 pound ham hocks, cracked
1/4 tsp. allspice or cumin
6 Jalapeño chilis, stems & seeds removed, chopped
2 medium onions, chopped
1 Tbs. parsley, chopped
1 Tbs. cilantro, chopped (opt.)
2 cloves garlic, minced
1 can (8 oz.) tomato sauce
1/2 cup dry red wine or 3 Tbs. lemon juice

      Rinse and sort beans, discarding any foreign material. Combine beans and water in a 5-quart pot and bring to a boil for 2 minutes. Cover and set aside for 1 hour. Drain off water and add the chicken broth, ham, allspice, chilis, onion, parsley, optional cilantro and garlic. Bring to a boil and reduce to a simmer. Cook for about 1 1/2 hours. Add the tomato sauce and simmer for 1/2 hour. Remove the ham and shred the meat. Puree the bean mixture, if desired, and add back to the pot. Add the ham and wine and reheat soup.

Salad of Swordfish
1 1/2 cups chicken stock
2 tsp. vinegar
3/4 pound swordfish, crosscut into 1/4-inch strips
1/2 cup celery, julienne
1/2 cup carrots, julienne
1/2 cup spring onions, sliced
1 Tbs. California diced green chilis (canned)
4 olives, sliced
1 Tbs. olive oil

1 Tbs. lemon juice
1 Tbs. orange juice
cayenne pepper
alfalfa sprouts or spinach leaves

Combine the chicken stock and vinegar in a large nonstick skillet. Bring to a boil, then simmer. Drop in fish and poach for 3 to 5 minutes. Remove fish and set aside. Now poach celery and carrots for 3 to 5 minutes. Drain and add the vegetables to the fish. Chill for 30 minutes.

Combine the rest of the ingredients except the cayenne and sprouts and add to the chilled fish. Coat evenly. Serve on the sprouts. Sprinkle with the cayenne pepper.

Tangy Crab Salad
Salad:
Mixed salad greens
1 small onion, thinly sliced
1 carrot, peeled and grated
3/4 pound cooked crabmeat
1 tomato, chopped
8 black olives, sliced
Dressing:
4 green Mexican chilis, roasted, peeled, seeded and chopped.
1/2 cup plain yogurt
2 Tbs. lime juice
1 tsp. horseradish sauce (opt.)

Combine the ingredients for the dressing. Refrigerate for an hour. Arrange the salad greens on 4 individual plates and arrange the onions and carrots on top. Next add the crab. Top with the tomatoes and olives. Serve the dressing on the side.

USING CHILIS WITH EGGS

Huevos Rancheros
Eggs, fried
corn or flour tortillas
mild salsa, warmed
avocado slices
chopped green onion
grated cheese

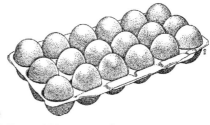

     Fry eggs and place on warmed tortillas. Pour 1/8 to 1/4 cup salsa over eggs and garnish with the avocado and onion. Sprinkle with cheese.

Mexican Omelet
butter or spray vegetable oil
2 eggs, beaten
1 Tbs. olives, chopped
1 Tbs. canned green chilis
1/2 Tbs. onion, minced

     Melt a bit of butter or spray a frying pan with oil. Add all the ingredients into the frying pan. As soon as the bottom begins to set, lift edges to let uncooked portion flow into contact with center of the pan. When eggs are set, turn omelet out of pan.

Potato Omelet
2 potatoes, peeled and diced
1 onion, diced
2 tsp. ground chili
1 tsp. butter
1 Tbs. canola oil
1 4 oz. can diced green chili
6 eggs

2 Tbs. water
1 tsp. parsley
1/2 tsp. salt

Saute potatoes, onion and chili powder in the butter and oil over medium heat. Cover and cook for fifteen minutes or until potatoes are tender. Add the green chilis. Combine the eggs, water, parsley and salt in a bowl and beat with a fork. Pour over the potato mixture in the skillet and cook over low heat until eggs are set.

Egg Burrito
1 medium onion, diced
1 clove garlic, minced
1 Tbs. canola oil
6 eggs, beaten
1/2 cup salsa
warmed flour tortillas
6 olives, sliced
2/3 cup grated cheese
1 small tomato, diced
1 small avocado, diced
sour cream
salt to taste

Saute onion and garlic in the oil until soft. Add the eggs and salsa. Scramble until done. Place some of the egg mixture in a tortilla and add some of the rest of the ingredients to taste. Roll into a burrito.

USING CHILIS IN ENTREES

Jambalaya
1 Tbs. canola oil
1/2 pound chicken, diced
1 onion, diced
1/2 pound smoked sausage
3 cloves garlic, minced
1 bay leaf
1 Tbs. parsley, minced
1/4 tsp. dried thyme
1/4 tsp. dried basil
1/4 tsp. ground cloves
1/4 tsp. ground anise, (opt.)
1/4 tsp. Cajun powder
1 1/2 cups chicken broth
3/4 cup rice
3 small hot red chilis, crushed
1/2 tsp. Louisiana hot sauce
Salt and pepper to taste

In a large pot, saute the onion and chicken until the onion is soft. Add the next 9 ingredients in oil and cook for an additional 5 minutes. Add the broth and bring to a boil. Boil for 5 minutes, then add the rest of the ingredients. Boil, then simmer, uncovered, until rice absorbs the liquid and is soft, about 15 to 20 minutes.

Casserole Enchilada
8 corn tortillas
canola oil
1 can (7 oz.) green chili salsa, heated
4 eggs, separated
1 Tbs. whole wheat flour
6 oz. shredded jack cheese

3 canned California green chilis, seeds removed and chopped

Fry the tortillas in a frying pan brushed with oil and dip in heated chili salsa. Put 1 tortilla in bottom of a 7 or 8-inch baking dish (2 inches deep at least) that has been lightly sprayed with vegetable oil. Arrange remaining tortillas, overlapping, around sides and slightly over bottom center tortilla. Beat egg whites until stiff. With same beater whip egg yolks until slightly thickened. Beat in the flour. Stir in 2/3 of the cheese, chilis and egg white. Pour into dish with tortillas. Fold tortillas down over filling. Spoon remaining salsa over tortillas, then sprinkle with cheese. Bake uncovered in a 375 degree oven for 30 minutes.

Indian Spice Chicken
4 spring onions, sliced
1 Tbs. canola oil
10 whole cardamon pods, crushed
1/4 tsp. ground cumin
1/4 tsp. lemon peel, diced fine
1/4 tsp. ground cloves
1/4 tsp. cinnamon
1 tsp. ginger, minced
3 dried red chilis, stems & seeds removed, crushed
1 tsp. honey
2 cups water
1 whole chicken, cleaned
salt to taste

Saute the onion in oil in a pot and add the cardamon and toast for one minute. Stir in all the seasonings and add the water. Stir and bring to a boil. Add the chicken and cover. Simmer for 45 minutes, turning the chicken 3 times. Remove the cover and cook until the the chicken is done, turning often to coat the chicken with the spices.

Apricot Chicken
2 tsp. cornstarch
2 tsp. apple juice or water
1/2 pound chicken breast, cut into strips
1 tsp. ginger, minced
2 tsp. garlic, minced
1 Tbs. white wine
2 Tbs. soy sauce
1 Tbs. hot bean sauce
5 dried apricots,cut in pieces and soaked in the wine
1 1/2 tsp. honey
1 Tbs. canola oil
5 small dried hot chilis

Combine the cornstarch and apple juice. Toss with the chicken in a zip lock bag and marinate for 15 minutes. Mix together the rest of the ingredients except the oil and chilis, then set aside. This will be the sauce. Heat a wok until hot and add the oil. As soon as the oil is hot, add the chilis and chicken. Stir-fry until chicken is almost done and add the sauce. Cook for another 45 seconds. Serve on top of cooked brown rice.

Turkey Treat
1/2 medium size onion, finely chopped
2 tsp. finely chopped almonds
1 Tbs. olive oil
1 can (10 oz.) tomatillos
1/2 Tbs. cilantro, minced

1 1/2 Tbs. minced canned
California green chilis,
seeds removed
1 cup chicken broth
1 pound sliced cooked
turkey
3 cups hot cooked wild
rice or brown rice

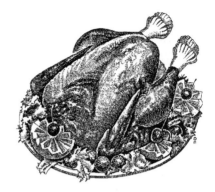

Combine the onion,
almonds, and oil in a pan
over medium heat and cook, stirring, until onion is limp.
Whirl tomatillos and their liquid in a blender until mixture
is fairly smooth (or rub through wire strainer, using all
liquid and pulp). Add to the onion mixture. Stir in cilantro
and chilis. Add the chicken broth and boil rapidly, uncovered, until reduced to about 1 1/4 cups. Stir occasionally.

Arrange meat in a wide frying pan. Pour sauce
over the meat and cover. Warm over low heat until
mixture begins to bubble slightly. Simmer for 5 to 10
minutes. Add salt to taste and serve on top of the rice.

Chilis Rellenos
8 fresh California chilis, peeled or
1 can (7 oz) California green chilis
1/4 cup almonds, slivered
1/2 Tbs. butter
1/2 pound lean ground beef
1 Tbs. onion, minced fine
1 clove garlic, minced fine
1/4 cup tomato puree
1/4 cup raisins
2 Tbs. dry sherry
1 tsp. ground cinnamon

1/2 tsp. salt
1/4 tsp. ground cloves
1/8 tsp. allspice
1 Tbs. vinegar
1 Tbs. dry sherry
1 tsp. fructose
4 eggs
4 Tbs. whole wheat flour
1 Tbs. water
1/4 tsp. salt
butter

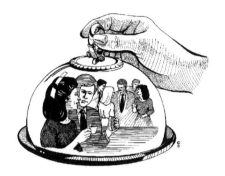

Drain the can chilis and slit down the side of each. Remove the seeds. Do the same for fresh chilis after peeling them.

Make the filling by lightly toasting the almond in the butter in a frying pan. Remove the almonds and brown the beef and onion. Add the garlic, tomato, raisins, sherry, the spices, vinegar, sherry and fructose. Cook, uncovered, until liquid is almost all gone.

Stuff the chilis. Fold the edges over each other to hold in the filling, which includes almonds. Roll each chili in flour to coat all over.

Separate the eggs. Beat whites until they form soft peaks. Beat yolks with the 4 Tbs. flour, water and salt. Fold into whites.

Over medium heat, melt enough butter to coat bottom of frying pan. Make an oval mound of about 1/2 cup of the egg mixture. Quickly lay a stuffed chili in the center of the mound and spoon about 1/3 cup mixture over top of chili. Cook for 2 to 3 minutes; gently turn and cook for 3 minutes longer or until golden brown.

You can use a cheese filling by stuffing each chili with a piece of jack cheese one inch shorter than the chili.

Enchilada Pie
1 pound lean ground beef
1 onion, chopped
1 clove garlic, minced
1 tsp. salt
1/4 tsp. cumin powder
1 Tbs. chili powder
1 can (8 oz.) tomato sauce
6 corn tortillas
olive oil
1 can (4 1/2 oz.) black olives, chopped
1 cup Cheddar cheese, grated
1/3 cup water
Brown beef and onion in a frying pan. Add the garlic, salt, cumin powder, chili powder, and tomato sauce. Spread each tortilla with a touch of oil and alternate layers of tortillas, meat sauce, olives and cheese in a 2-quart casserole dish. Add water. Cover and bake in a 400 degree oven for 20 minutes.

Green Chili Stew
2 pounds boneless beef chuck, cut in 1-inch cubes
2 Tbs. olive oil
1 bell pepper diced
1 medium onion, diced
2 cloves garlic, minced
2 cans (1 lb. 12 oz. each) tomatoes
1 can (7 oz.) California green chilis, seeded and chopped
1/4 cup parsley, chopped
1/2 tsp. honey

1/4 tsp. ground cloves
2 tsp. ground cumin
1 tsp. lemon juice
1 cup red wine or beef broth
Salt to taste

Brown the meat in 2 Tbs olive oil on all sides in a large frying pan. Remove meat with a slotted spoon and set aside. Throw away drippings, add the olive oil and cook the bell pepper, onion, and garlic until soft. In a large pot, pour in the tomatoes with the liquid. Break up tomatoes with a spoon. Add the chilis, parsley, honey, cloves, cumin, lemon juice and wine. Bring to a boil, then reduce heat to a simmer. Add all of the ingredients together, cover, and cook over low heat for 1 1/2 hours, stirring occasionally. Remove cover and simmer for 1 more hour or until meat is tender.

Chili
1 large onion, diced
1 celery stock, diced
3 cloves garlic, minced
2 jalapenos, stemmed & seeded, minced
1 1/2 pounds lean ground beef
1/2 Tbs. canola oil
1 (7-ounce) can diced green chilis
2 to 3 Tbs. chili
powder
1 can (16 ounces)
whole tomatoes
3 Tbs. tomato paste
2 tsp. ground cumin
1 1/2 cups water
1 bay leaf
1/2 tsp. Worcester
sauce (opt.)

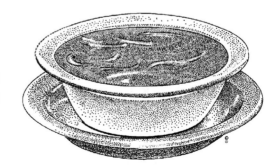

1 tsp. sugar
6 ounces beer
salt and pepper to taste

In a large pot, saute the onions, celery, garlic and jalapeno in the oil. Add the beef and cook until meat is brown. Add remaining ingredients. Mash the tomatoes in the sauce. Simmer for 1 1/2 to 2 hours, stirring occasionally.

Stuffed Beef Steaks
5 Anaheim chilis
4 jalapeno chilis
1 medium onion, chopped
3 cloves garlic, minced
1 Tbs. olive oil
1/2 Tbs. parsley, minced
1/2 grated Monterey Jack cheese
2 pounds trimmed filet of beef, cut in 4 thick steaks
fresh ground pepper (opt.)

Remove the stems and seeds, then chop the chilis. Saute the onion, chilis, and garlic in the oil until slightly soft. Remove, cool and mix in the cheese and parsley. Refrigerate this a day before using it.

Slice into the steaks from the edge, creating a pocket for the stuffing. Stuff with the chili mixture and close the opening with a toothpick. You can season the outside of the steaks with the black pepper. Grill over hot charcoal or gas barbecue.

Hot Time Halibut
1/4 cup hot pepper sauce
1/4 cup red wine vinegar
1 Tbs. olive oil
1/2 Tbs. Worcestershire sauce
1/4 tsp. garlic powder

2 Tbs. smoke-flavor BBQ sauce
4 halibut steaks
In a small bowl, blend the first 6 ingredients. Place this marinade in a zip lock bag with the fish and gently coat the fish with the marinade. Refrigerate for several hours. Place the fish on a nonstick baking sheet and bake in a 425 degree oven for 10-15 minutes until done.

Tuna Cakes
2 slices whole wheat bread (crusts removed)
1 can (6 1/2 ounces) tuna, drained
1 egg
1 pimiento, chopped
1/4 tsp. celery salt
1/8 tsp. cayenne pepper
1/4 tsp. lemon juice
1 Tbs. canned California diced green chilis
Tear the bread into small pieces. Mix all the ingredients together in a bowl. Shape the mixture into 3 firm patties about 1/2 inch thick. Fry the patties in oil over medium heat until golden brown on both sides, 4 to 5 minutes.

Scallops in a Blanket
1/4 cup spring onions, sliced
1/4 cup olives, sliced
1 clove garlic, minced
1 tsp. chili peppers, minced
1/8 tsp. ground cumin
1 pound scallops
4 flour tortillas (9 or 10 inch)
1/2 cup chunky salsa
1/2 cup no-fat sour cream

Saute the onions, olives, garlic and chili in oil in a frying pan for 2 minutes over medium heat. Add the cumin and scallops and saute for 3 minutes. Warm the tortillas in a cloth napkin in the microwave for 20-25 seconds. Spoon the scallop mixture onto the tortillas, then roll to wrap and fold under ends. Serve with the salsa and sour cream.

Hog Heaven
16 dried New Mexican chilis, stems removed
2 1/2 cups water
4 cloves garlic
1 tsp. dried oregano
1/2 tsp. dried basil
1 tsp. dried parsley
1/2 cup light white wine
3 pounds lean pork, cut into strips

Cover the chilis with the water and simmer for 10 minutes or until softened. Place the drained chilis and seasonings in a blender and puree with just enough of the wine to make a thick sauce. Marinate the pork in the sauce overnight.

In a 300 degree preheated oven, bake the pork in the marinade, covered, for a couple of hours or until the meat is very tender and starts to fall apart. Uncover during the last 30 minutes of cooking to slowly bake off excess liquid.

Chipotle Tenderloin
3 dried or canned chipotle chilis
6 cloves garlic
1 small onion, chopped
1/2 tsp. ground allspice
1/2 tsp. ground mace

1/2 tsp. ground cloves
1/4 cup vinegar
1/2 cup orange juice
1/4 cup lime juice
1/4 cup sucanat or brown sugar
1/2 tsp. black pepper
1 cup olive oil
2 pork tenderloins, trimmed of excess fat

If using dried chipotles, cover with hot water for 15 minutes to soften. Remove the stems. Place all ingredients except the oil and meat in a blender and puree while slowly drizzling in the oil. Place the meat and this marinate in a ziplock bag for at least an hour.

Bake in a 400 degree oven for about 8 minutes, turning every 2 minutes. Slice the tenderloins into 1/2 inch pieces and serve.

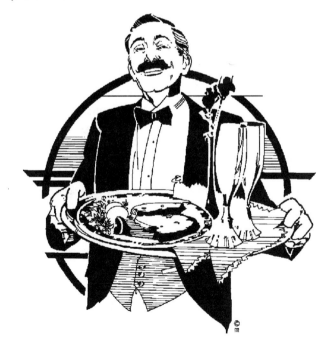

APPENDIX

WHERE TO FIND HOT CHILI PRODUCTS

Mail-Order Catalogs

Arizona Pepper Products
PO Box 40605
Mesa AZ 85210
800-359-3912
www.azgunslinger.com

Calido Chile Traders
1361 Roelke Dr
South Bend IN 46614
888-243-1821
www.calido-indiana.com

Chile Hill Emporium
Box 9100
Bernalillo NM 87004
505-867-3294

Chile Pepper Magazine
1701 River Run Suite # 901
Fort Worth TX 76107
800-ZESTY-ME
www.chilepepper.com

The Chile Shop
109 East Water St
Santa Fe NM 87501
505-983-6080
www.thechileshop.com

Chile Today, Hot Tomale
31 Rich Boynton Rd
Dover NJ 07801
800-HOT-PEPPER
www.chiletoday.com

Chili Pepper Emporium
901 Rio Grande NW Suite A-194
Albuquerque NM 87104
800-288-9648
www.chilepepperemporium.com

Chili's Fire Pit
9570 Mentor Ave
Mentor OH 44060
440-352-8058
www.chilisfirepit.com

ColoradoSmokeHouse.com, Inc.
PO Box 1352
Berthoud CO 80513
800-675-4869
www.imapepperhead.com

The Cook's Garden
PO Box 1889
Southampton PA 18966-0895
800-457-9703
www.cooksgarden.com

Cosmic Chile
1612 Gold Ave
Bozeman MT 59715
800-955-9724
www.cosmicchile.com

Dat'l Do-It
3255 Parker Dr
St Augustine FL 32084
800-HOT-DATL
www.datldoit.com

Enchanted Seeds
PO Box 6087
Las Cruces NM 88006
505-233-3033
www.enchantedseeds.com

Fiery Foods & BBQ Magazine
800-352-8039
www.fiery-foods.com

Figueroa Brothers
922 Industry Rd
Kenner LA 70062
800-886-6354
www.hotsaucezone.com

Flamingo Flats
Box 441
St Michaels MD 21663
800-468-8841
www.flamingoflats.com

Frieda's
Los Alamitos CA 90720
800-421-9477
www.friedas.com

Gil's Gourmet Gallery
577 Ortiz Ave
Sand City CA 93955
800-438-7480
www.gilsgourmet.com

GMB Specialty Foods
PO Box 962
San Juan Capistrano CA 92693-0962
800-809-8298
www.gmb-foods.com

Golden Grille
2805 Division St Suite 102
Metairie LA 70002
504-780-0830
www.goldengrille.com

Gypsy Kitchen
1241 Hancock St
Quincy MA 02169
617-227-9649
www.drhot.net

Hatch Chile Express
PO Box 350
Hatch NM 87937
800-292-4454
www.hatch-chile.com

Hot Licks
Seaport Village
865 West Harbor Dr
San Diego CA 92126
619-235-4000
www.2hotlicks.com

Hot Papa's
Round Rock TX 78681-5652
512-388-3258
www.hotpapas.com

HotSauce.com, Inc.
PO Box 801933
Miami FL 33280
954-929-3289
www.hotsauce.com

Hot Sauce Harry's
10606 Shady Trail Suite 20
Dallas TX 75220
800-588-8979
www.hotsauceharrys.com

Hot Hot Hot
305 North Beacon
San Pedro CA 90731
800-959-7742
www.hothothot.com

Jones and Bones
621 Capitola Ave
Capitola CA 95010
831-462-0521
www.jonesandbones.com

Melissa's World Variety Produce
PO Box 21127
Los Angeles CA 90021
800-588-0151
www.melissas.com

Mo Hotta, Mo Betta
PO Box 1026
Savannah GA 31402
800-462-3220
www.mohotta.com

Native Seeds
526 N 4th Ave
Tucson AZ 85705-8450
520-620-5561
www.nativeseeds.org

New Orleans School of Cooking
524 Saint Louis St
New Orleans LA 70130
504-525-2665
www.nosoc.com

Pendery's
1221 Manufacturing St
Dallas TX 75207
800-533-1870
www.penderys.com

The Pepper Gal
PO Box 23006
Fort Lauderdale FL 33311
954-537-5540
www.peppergal.com

Pepper Joe's
7 Tyburn Court
Timonium MD 21093
Fax 410-628-0507
www.pepperjoe.com

Peppers
Rehoboth Outlets # 3
1815 Ocean Outlets
Rehoboth Beach DE 19971
800-998-FIRE
www.peppers.com

Pete's Pepper Palace
Village Square
418 Pearl Street
Burlington ON L7R 2N1 Canada
888-343-9994
www.iloveithot.com

Plants of the Southwest
3095 Agua Fria Rd
Santa Fe NM 87507
800-788-SEED
www.plantsofthesouthwest.com

Redwood City Seed Co
PO Box 361
Redwood City CA 94064
650-325-SEED
www.batnet.com/rwc-seed

Reimer Seeds
PO Box 236
Mount Holly NC 28120-0236
Fax 704-544-3762
www.reimerseeds.com

Renee's Garden Seeds
7389 W Zayante Rd
Felton CA 95018
888-880-7228
www.reneesgarden.com

Salas Express
PO Box 1157
Fredericksburg TX 78624
800-437-2572
www.salasexpress.com

Salsas, Etc!
421 Center St
Yuba City CA 95991
800-987-8512
www.salsasetc.com

Sambet's Cajun Store
8650 Spicewood Springs Rd
Austin TX 78759
800-472-6238

Santa Cruz Chili & Spice Co
PO Box 177
Tumacacori AZ 85640
520-398-2591
www.santacruzchili.com

Santa Fe School of Cooking
116 W San Francisco St
Santa Fe NM 87501
800-982-4688
www.santafeschoolofcooking.com

Santa Fe Seasons
1590 San Mateo Lane
Santa Fe NM 87505
800-264-5535
www.santafeseasons.com

Seed Savers Exchange
3076 North Winn Road
Decorah IA 52102
www.seedsavers.org

Seeds of Change
PO Box 15700
Santa Fe NM 87507
888-762-SEED
www.seedsofchange.com

A Southern Season
Highway 15-501 at Estes Drive
University Mall
Chapel Hill NC 27514
800-253-3663
www.southernseason.com

Sunny Caribbee Spice Co
PO Box 3237
St Thomas VDA
US Virgin Islands 00803
284-494-2178
www.sunnycarribbee.com

Tabasco Country Store
McIlhenny Company
Avery Island LA 70513
880-TABASCO-1
www.countrystore.tabasco.com

Terra Time and Tide
590 E 59th ST
Jacksonville FL 32208
904-764-0376
www.pepperhot.com

Try a New Sauce
PO Box 341
Hudson NH 03051
877-292-4731
www.tryanewsauce.com

Twilley Seed Co Inc
121 Gary Road
Hodges SC 29653
800-622-SEED
www.twilleyseed.com

Uncle Steve's Hot Stuff
Fredericksburg VA
www.ushotstuff.com

Whole Earth Grainery
111 Ivinson Ave
Laramie WY 82070
307-745-4268

✂ please cut here

The Healing Power of

Cayenne Pepper

Complete Handbook of Cayenne Home Remedies

Patrick Quillin, PhD, RD, CNS

Cayenne Pepper Book

90-Day Money-Back Guarantee

☐ **YES!** Please rush _____ additional copies of the *Cayenne Pepper Book* and my FREE copy of the bonus booklet *"Use It Or Lose It - Home Remedies For Your Mind"* for only $12.95 plus $3.98 postage & handling. I understand that I must be completely satisfied or I can return it within 90 days for a full and prompt refund of my purchase price. The FREE gift is mine to keep regardless. Want to save even more? Do a favor for a close relative or friend and order two books for only $13.86 postpaid. That's 2 for only $20 postpaid.

I am enclosing $ _____ by: ☐ Check ☐ Money Order (Make checks payable to James Direct, Inc.)

Charge my credit card Signature _____

☐ VISA ☐ MasterCard ☐ DISCOVER ☐ AMEX

Card No. _____ Exp. date _____

Name _____

Address _____

City _____ State _____ Zip _____

Mail To: JAMES DIRECT, INC. • 1459 South Main Street, Box 3093, Dept. CP106 N. Canton, Ohio 44720 • http://www.jamesdirect.com

✂ please cut here

Use this coupon to order the "The Healing Power of Cayenne Pepper Book" for a friend or family member -- or copy the ordering information onto a plain piece of paper and mail to:

The Healing Power of Cayenne Pepper
Dept. CP106
1459 South Main Street
Box 3093
N. Canton, Ohio 44720

Preferred Customer Reorder Form

Order this...	If you want a book on...	Cost...	Number of Copies...
Emily's Vinegar Diet Book	This is the easy-to-follow diet you have been waiting for! It helps you lose weight without counting calories or being hungry. This time, you'll keep the weight off-for life!	$9.95	
American Cookery	Discovered in the archives, here is the very first cookbook published in America by an American author. Wonderful historic collection!	$9.95	
Amish Gardening Secrets	You too can learn the special gardening secrets the Amish use to produce huge tomato plants and bountiful harvests. Information packed 800-plus collection for you to tinker with and enjoy.	$9.95	
The Food Remedy Handbook	*Big 208 Page Book!* In "The Food Remedy Handbook" you'll discover the secret power of blueberries, lemon, cinnamon and other ordinary foods. *And Much More!*	$9.95	
The Vinegar Book II	What else can vinegar be used for? PLENTY! This book gives you even more new and exciting ways to use vinegar for good health and natural healing. Discover how the combination of vinegar, honey & garlic can help relieve the pain of arthritis, reduce cholesterol, fight cancer, assist weight loss and MUCH MORE!	$9.95	
The Vinegar Home Guide	Learn how to clean and freshen with natural, environmentally-safe vinegar in the house, garden and laundry. Plus, delicious home-style recipes!	$9.95	
Hydrogen Peroxide	In *The Amazing Health and Household Uses of Hydrogen Peroxide* you'll get kitchen hints, health tips and skin tonics using that common medicine cabinet staple – hydrogen peroxide!	$9.95	

Any combination of the above $9.95 items qualifies for the following discounts...

		Total NUMBER of $9.95 items	

Order any 2 items for: $15.95	Order any 4 items for: $24.95	Order any 6 items for: $34.95 and receive 7th item FREE	Any additional items for: $5 each
Order any 3 items for: $19.95	Order any 5 items for: $29.95		

		Total COST of $9.95 items	

Order this...	If you want a book on...	Cost	Copies
Coconut Cures	Learn coconut's role in the fight against diabetes & heart disease as well as health tips to increase energy, help with weight control as well as remedies for fever blisters, candida, varicose veins, gum disease and more.	$12.95	
~~NEW~~ **Vinegar & Tea Book**	The first book in a brand new series! Explores the benefits of two of the healthiest liquids around: tea and vinegar. Blending the two may be the best thing you can add to your diet to stay healthy! Over 801 tonics and super remedies.	$19.95	
The Vinegar Anniversary Book	Completely updated with the latest research and brand new remedies and uses for apple cider vinegar. Handsome coffee table collector's edition you'll be proud to display. *Big 232-page book!*	$19.95	

	Postage & Handling	$3.98*
	TOTAL	

90-DAY MONEY-BACK GUARANTEE

* order 10 or more books, $6.96

Please rush me the items marked above. I understand that I must be completely satisfied or I can return any item within 90 days with proof of purchase for a full and prompt refund of my purchase price.

I am enclosing $_____ by: ❑ Check ❑ Money Order (Make checks payable to James Direct Inc)

VISA MasterCard DISCOVER AMEX

Charge my credit card Signature _____

Card No. _____ Exp. Date _____

Name _____ Address _____

City _____ State _____ Zip _____

Telephone Number (_____) _____

❑ Yes! I'd like to know about freebies, specials and new products before they are nationally advertised.

My email address is: _____

Mail To: **James Direct Inc.** • 1459 S. Main St., Box 3093, Dept. A1058 • N. Canton, Ohio 44720
Customer Service (330) 494-5053 • *http://www.jamesdirect.com*

EMILY'S VINEGAR DIET BOOK

This easiest diet ever helps you lose pounds and inches, and keep them off! With a tonic of apple cider vinegar and honey there is no confusing calorie counting, food restrictions or expensive supplements. Increase your energy level while the pounds melt away. See how to use the "magic" thermogenesis to be thinner, look younger and feel more vigorous -- without depriving yourself of the foods you love!

AMERICAN COOKERY

In 1796 Amelia Simmons published what would become the "mother of all cookbooks" and two original copies are known to exist...one in the Bitting Collection of the Library of Congress, the other in the Whitney Collection of the New York Public Library. By special permission, this Ohio publisher has a facsimile copy available for a limited time...

AMISH GARDENING SECRETS

There's something for everyone in *Amish Gardening Secrets.* This BIG collection contains over 800 gardening hints, suggestions, time savers and tonics that have been passed down over the years in Amish communities and elsewhere.

THE FOOD REMEDY HANDBOOK

The Food Remedy Handbook is full of natural cures as well as painless organization techniques and time and money-saving tips that are sure to save you untold amounts of cash!

THE VINEGAR BOOK II

You asked for it — Emily Thacker delivered! Still more ways to use vinegar – around the house – for your pets – in the medicine cabinet and some surprising vinegar facts! There's even good news on Vinegar's role in the fight against aging!

THE VINEGAR HOME GUIDE

Emily Thacker presents her second volume of hundreds of all-new vinegar tips. Use versatile vinegar to add a low-sodium zap of flavor to your cooking, as well as getting your house "white-glove" clean for just pennies. Plus, safe and easy tips on shining and polishing brass, copper & pewter and removing stubborn stains & static cling in your laundry!

THE AMAZING HEALTH AND HOUSEHOLD USES OF HYDROGEN PEROXIDE

Find out how to use hydrogen peroxide to kill bacteria, ease arthritis pain, reduce age spots and much more!

COCONUT CURES

Why are they calling Coconut Oil the Cure for All Illness? Within this 256-page book you'll find out it's 1000 uses and why it's been the best kept health secret in the USA!

NEW ---

VINEGAR & TEA BOOK

Tea along with apple cider vinegar may be a wonder elixir for good health! Over 801 old-time tea and vinegar tonics and tried and true remedies and recipes in this amazing collector's edition.

THE VINEGAR ANNIVERSARY BOOK

Handsome coffee table edition and brand new information on Mother Nature's Secret Weapon – apple cider vinegar!

* Each Book has its own FREE Bonus!

> All these important books carry our NO-RISK GUARANTEE. Enjoy them for three full months. If you are not 100% satisfied simply return the book(s) along with proof of purchase, for a prompt, "no questions asked" refund!